W9-DIS-664

HEADACHE
RELIEF FOR
WOMEN

*Also by Alan M. Rapoport, M.D.,
and Fred D. Sheftell, M.D.*

HEADACHE RELIEF
CONQUERING HEADACHE

HEADACHE RELIEF FOR WOMEN

How You Can Manage
and Prevent Pain

ALAN M. RAPOPORT, M.D.,
AND FRED D. SHEFTELL, M.D.

LITTLE, BROWN AND COMPANY
Boston · New York · Toronto · London

COPYRIGHT © 1995 BY ALAN M. RAPOPORT AND FRED D. SHEFTELL

ALL RIGHTS RESERVED. NO PART OF THIS BOOK MAY BE REPRO-
DUCED IN ANY FORM OR BY ANY ELECTRONIC OR MECHANICAL
MEANS, INCLUDING INFORMATION STORAGE AND RETRIEVAL SYS-
TEMS, WITHOUT PERMISSION IN WRITING FROM THE PUBLISHER,
EXCEPT BY A REVIEWER WHO MAY QUOTE BRIEF PASSAGES IN A
REVIEW.

FIRST EDITION

*This book is not intended to replace medical care under the direct
supervision of a qualified physician. Before embarking on any changes in
your health regimen, consult your physician.*

LIBRARY OF CONGRESS CATALOGING-IN-PUBLICATION DATA
Rapoport, Alan M.
    Headache relief for women : how you can manage and prevent
pain / Alan M. Rapoport and Fred D. Sheftell. — 1st ed.
        p.   cm.
    ISBN 0-316-73393-8 (HC)
    ISBN 0-316-73391-1 (PB)
    1. Headache.   2. Women—Diseases.   3. Migraine.   4. Headache —
Endocrine aspects. I. Sheftell, Fred D. II Title.
RC392.R36   1995
616.8'491'0082 — dc20   95-6757

10 9 8 7 6 5 4 3 2 1

MV-NY

Designed by Jeanne Abboud

Published simultaneously in Canada by Little, Brown & Company (Canada) Limited
PRINTED IN THE UNITED STATES OF AMERICA

To all women who have suffered with headache. Trust yourselves and take an active role in your treatment. Take heart . . . you don't have to "learn to live with it."

To our families. Thank you for your support and encouragement and for being there. To our colleagues, for their efforts in helping others and teaching us.

AR
FS

CONTENTS

We wish to thank Betsy Ryan, president of Bascom Communications, who produced this book with care and intelligence. Many thanks also to Rachel Krany, a gifted writer and Jennifer Josephy, a gifted editor. Thanks also to Stephen Lamont for the meticulous professionalism he brought to this manuscript.

HEADACHE
RELIEF FOR
WOMEN

CHAPTER 1

Taking Responsibility

"Oh, it's just a little headache — what's the big deal?"
"Can't you just take an aspirin and forget about it?"
"You get headaches? You must have a really hard time handling your feelings!"
"Another headache? You're just trying to get out of visiting my mother!"

I F YOU SUFFER FROM RECURRENT HEADACHE, you're probably all too familiar with statements like these. Although you're among the more than 20 percent of all Americans who are afflicted with migraine and other severe headache, very likely your problem has not been recognized or taken seriously — by your friends and family, by your coworkers, by your health care providers, perhaps not even by you yourself. Small wonder, for despite its widespread incidence and crippling effects, this painful problem has yet to gain general acceptance as a valid medical disorder.

Migraine gives some people mild hallucinations, temporarily blinds others, shows up not only as a headache but as a gastrointestinal disturbance, a painful sensitivity to all sensory stimuli, an abrupt overpowering fatigue, a strokelike aphasia, and a crippling inability to make even the most routine connections. . . . The actual headache, when it comes, brings with it chills, sweating, nausea, a debility that seems to stretch the very limits of endurance. That no one dies of migraine seems, to someone deep into an attack, an ambiguous blessing. . . .

"Why not take a couple of aspirin," the unafflicted will say from the doorway. . . . All of us who have migraine suffer not only from the attacks themselves but from this common conviction that we are perversely refusing to cure ourselves by taking a couple of aspirin, that we are making ourselves sick, that we "bring it on ourselves."

JOAN DIDION, "IN BED," *THE WHITE ALBUM*

Some 23 million women and 8 million men in America suffer from migraine, a particularly painful and disabling form of headache. Yet migraineurs frequently think of themselves as special cases, alone in their suffering — and in their inability to control the profoundly painful and disruptive effects of their "little headaches." Many people who suffer from migraine, as well as those who experience tension-type headache, don't see themselves as afflicted by a common, understandable, and treatable disorder. Instead, they blame themselves, believing that if they were stronger, more emotionally healthy, or somehow "better people," their headaches would not be so severe.

Migraine is especially problematic for women, both because the vast majority of migraineurs are women (after puberty, women with migraine outnumber their male counterparts by almost three to one) and because in our society, women's health complaints have a tendency to be dismissed, ignored, or trivialized — by doctors, by friends and family, and by women themselves. According to one study, between 25 and 29 percent of all women get a migraine at least once in their lives. Another widely accepted conservative study found that 17.6 percent of all women suffer from migraine. Yet 60 percent of all migraine sufferers — most of whom are women — are not in treatment. Either they themselves don't recognize the legitimacy of their complaint, or their physicians do not grasp the seriousness of the problem.

This widespread ignorance about headache is particularly distressing when we consider that the problem is becoming ever more serious. According to one study, from 1980 to 1989 there was a 77 percent increase in the prevalence of migraine in patients under the age of forty-five. Migraine and other types of headache are continuing to affect more and more women like the following:

> *G.G. is a thirty-three-year-old woman who has had headaches since the age of fifteen. Every month, just about the time she gets her period, she wakes up with a dull, hammering pain that increases in intensity over the next several hours, concentrated in the area around her right eye and temple. These headaches make G.G. nauseated, frequently causing her to vomit. When she has a headache, she can't bear bright light or loud sounds, and often her vision blurs. Most of the time, she is simply incapacitated, withdrawing to a dark room to sleep if she is lucky, to "ride out the pain" if she is not. Her headache will last the entire day — from twelve to twenty-four hours — leaving her exhausted and "washed out" for several more hours afterward.*

> *L.S. is a fourteen-year-old girl who has been having headaches since she was eight. She knows she's starting a headache when she gets a small blind spot off to the right, surrounded by a bright, glimmering border of light. Over the next twenty to thirty minutes, the blind spot gets larger, until she can't see at all. L.S. doesn't look forward to the recovery of her vision, however, because when the blind spot starts to shrink, her right temple begins to throb with a severe, pounding pain. The headache has begun — and it will last for eight to twelve hours. When L.S. has a headache, she can't eat and*

frequently is overcome by nausea, vomiting, and dizziness. She can't attend school, enjoy a conversation, or engage in any other daily activity. Instead, she lies in bed with the covers pulled over her head, trying not to move.

K.R. is a fifty-year-old woman who has been having tension headaches ever since she turned thirty-five. Her headaches are not considered migraines, but they are painful and disruptive nonetheless. Often, she says, her head will start to ache late in the morning, with a pain that increases as the day goes on. Unlike migraineurs, K.R. can continue to function with a headache, but its tight, viselike pain has become an all-too-frequent part of her life.

A.H. has been having headaches since she was seventeen. Now she's forty-three. Over the years her headaches have changed in quality, becoming an even-greater part of her daily life.

Even when she was younger, A.H.'s headaches used to "knock her out" completely. For eight to twelve hours, she'd be overwhelmed by a throbbing pain on one or both sides of her head, along with nausea, vomiting, diarrhea, and sensitivity to light and sound. A.H.'s headaches left her completely unable to function; and whenever she got one, she'd have to cancel all her activities for that day.

As she got older, A.H. found that her headaches were getting worse, lasting longer, and coming on more frequently. Finally, she was getting three to four attacks every month, with each headache lasting one or two days. To make matters worse, she was experiencing a constant, dull pain — like a "tight headband" — whenever she was not laid up with an incapacitating migraine. By the time she finally sought the help of headache special-

ists, A.H. was virtually never without some form of headache pain. Her "mixed headache syndrome"— migraine plus tension-type headache — did not respond to the previous medication she'd been given. Nor did they respond to biofeedback. All neurological tests turned up normal — yet A.H.'s headaches were dominating her life.

We know about women like G.G., L.S., K.R., and A.H. because they came to us for treatment. Millions more like them are not receiving treatment, but they too are suffering from migraine, tension-type, and "mixed" headache (also known as "chronic daily headache").

If you or someone you know is among the millions of women suffering from some form of headache, take heart. Painful and disabling though these headaches may be, they *can* be treated. They aren't caused by some mysterious character defect or by some flawed response to stress, but by electrical and biochemical processes in the brain. A wide variety of drug and nondrug treatments are available both to help prevent headaches from coming on and to minimize their effects if they do begin. And perhaps the best news of all is that *you* can be an active partner in your own treatment. Your behavior, your choices, and your attitudes can all make an enormous difference in your journey toward finding health and freeing yourself from pain.

MYTHS AND FACTS ABOUT HEADACHE

When patients first come to us for treatment, we sometimes have the impression that the myths about headache have proved almost as painful as the headaches themselves! Let's take a closer look at those myths, particularly as they affect women.

Myth: A person who has a headache isn't really suffering—it's just a little pain. "After all, I get headaches and it's not so terrible," says the long-suffering husband, lover, child, friend, or coworker. "I'm tired of Marge making such a big deal out of such a little thing. How bad can it be?"

Fact: Although some headaches are relatively minor sources of pain, many headaches, particularly migraines, are intensely painful. A person who has never had a truly bad headache—and some people never get one — cannot compare his or her experience of headache pain with that of the woman suffering from migraine or from a severe tension-type headache. It's like comparing a bruise on the arm to a compound fracture.

Sadly, many women choose to believe the judgments of those around them, rather than trusting in their own experience. Many women find it difficult to stick to their own opinions, particularly if their own ideas put them at odds with loved ones or people in authority. So although a woman with headache *knows* she's suffering, she may also worry that she's exaggerating.

Myth: Having a bad headache is just an excuse to get out of work or to spend a day in bed. "This is the fifth time that Julia has been out sick in the past three weeks," a coworker might fume. "And that's not counting the two days she had to leave early. I'm tired of covering for her. What is her problem?"

Fact: Many headaches — particularly migraines and cluster headaches — are in fact disabling. Migraine headaches are often accompanied by nausea and vomiting, chills and fever, disturbances of vision, and extreme sensitivity to light or sound. A person with a migraine may find that holding her head at a particular angle is excruciatingly painful or that she literally doesn't have the strength to walk across the room. People who have cluster headaches — more common among men, but occasionally experienced by women — have said that the pain is far worse than complicated childbirth or accidental amputation. Even so-called tension-type headaches may be accompanied by nausea or by pain sufficient to affect concentration.

If a woman is under pressure — from others, herself, or both — to put others' needs first, to be the "perfect mother," or to play a "superwoman" at home and at work, it may be particularly hard for her to accept her own limits. Thus, women are all too susceptible to the prevailing myth that they "don't need to" succumb to their headaches. And if a woman's headache does force her to leave work or to abandon household responsibilities, she may feel a profound sense of guilt about knuckling under to "such a little thing."

Myth: *A person who gets regular or disabling headaches is betraying a problem with her personality.* "I don't know what it is with Donna," Donna's mother might sigh. "Ever since she was a teenager, she's had these terrible headaches. I guess she just can't handle stress."

"I read that people with migraines have 'migraine personalities,'" Donna's sister might add. "They're supposed to be driven, compulsive perfectionists — just like Donna!"

Fact: *There is no correlation between any type of headache—including migraine — and any particular type of personality.* A person who is diagnosed with migraine, tension-type headache, or cluster headache is suffering from a chronic condition, like diabetes or arthritis. No studies have been able to turn up any correlation between diagnoses of chronic headache and particular personality traits.

The chronic condition of being headache-prone may cause a person to *translate* stress into headache, but that doesn't mean the person can't handle stress. It only means that her body reacts to stress in particular ways. Another person might translate stress into a stomachache, an ulcer, a backache, fatigue, or irritability. A headache-prone person translates it into headaches.

Why might a woman believe that her headaches reveal personality problems or problems with stress? Perhaps because women in today's society face a double bind, with the tacit message: If a woman doesn't work outside the home, she's not really accomplishing much of anything; but if she does work outside the home, she's neglecting her family or she's overly ambitious. Instead of blaming the society that has created this dilemma, a woman might be likely to blame herself for not being able to solve it. If a woman feels — even unconsciously — that she doesn't really "belong" in the workplace or that she isn't really "achieving" anything by staying at home, she may also feel that her headaches are the sign of the problem. If only she had a different personality! Then she would be happier at home or at work, and she wouldn't get headaches.

Likewise, women in positions of power or authority— positions that are inherently stressful — may feel doubly stressed by having to prove themselves or by having to handle more resentment and suspicion than would be directed at a man in the same position. A woman in such a circumstance may be all too ready to blame herself, both for the hard times she's having and for the headaches that seem inevitably to result. (For more about headache and emotions, see Chapter 8.)

Myth: A person who has been diagnosed with migraine or tension-type headache just has to grin and bear it; not much can be done about her condition. "I've been to three regular doctors and to a neurologist," Dolores might say. "At first, their pills worked fine, but sooner or later they always stopped working. I just don't think anyone can help me."

Fact: There are a wide range of drug and nondrug treatments that can be used both to prevent headaches and to ease the pain of the headaches that do occur. Unfortunately, many doctors are not knowledgeable about the latest discoveries in headache research. They may not take headache seriously as an ailment that causes enormous suffering — and as a condition that can be treated.

True, nothing can *cure* a woman who is headache-prone, at least not yet; she may continue to be susceptible to headache for many years to come. (Many people do experience spontaneous relief as they get older.) But there are many ways that a person and her doctor or health care provider can work together to make headache far less likely. There are also many ways to respond to the headaches that do come. No one who suffers from regular headache has to "grin and bear it" — it's just a matter of finding the right health care provider and working together to find the right treatment.

Myth: Headaches may be minor irritations, but when all is said and done, they aren't really a serious medical problem, like hypertension or heart disease. "All right, I understand that nobody likes having a headache," a doctor might say. "But after all, we're just talking about headaches here. There are plenty of far more serious diseases that warrant more of my attention."

Fact: In recent studies done on how headache affected people's quality of life, headache was found to interfere with normal functioning to a greater extent than almost any other chronic condition, including diabetes, arthritis, depression, and back problems. In an article in a 1994 edition of *PharmacoEconomics*, Glen D. Solomon reported on several studies that explored the relationship between headache and quality of life. The only chronic-condition patients whose functioning was as adversely affected as that of headache patients were people who had suffered myocardial infarction (heart attacks) within the past year and patients who suffered from congestive heart failure. The only disease state that had lower levels of patient well-being and functioning than headache was symptomatic HIV infection — in other words, AIDS.

Solomon fleshed out his gloomy summary with several disturbing examples. In one Canadian survey, for example, researchers found that nearly one-half of respondents with migraine discontinued their normal activities; nearly one-third required bed rest during their migraines. An American research team led by Jane T. Osterhaus found in 1992 that 55 percent of the migraineurs studied missed two workdays per month, while 88 percent worked 5.6 days per month at lower productivity due to migraine symptoms. As Solomon summarized the data, people suffering from migraine were the most likely to have problems maintaining their performance at work, while those with chronic daily headache (a kind of tension-type headache that may be related to migraine, see below) experienced mental health problems and a general impairment in functioning.

If we wanted to reduce the quality-of-life issue to dollars and cents, we could point to figures from the National Health Interview Survey and the Bureau of Labor Statistics showing that headache costs U.S. workers $1.3 billion in lost wages each year, while migraine results in 5.7 million days of restricted workplace activity per year, including over 3 million days spent bedridden. Since women are far more susceptible to migraine than men, 82 percent of that lost productivity is from women. And housewives suffer 3.2 million days of restricted activity annually. Altogether, according to Solomon, the U.S. economy loses $17.2 billion per year from "headache loss."

However, more than by the economic statistics, we are concerned by the thought of so many millions of headache sufferers getting improper treatment — or no treatment at all. (Remember, well over 50 percent of all migraineurs are not getting treatment, and the percentage for tension-type headache sufferers is even higher.) While a certain amount of suffering from headache may be inevitable for some people, a great deal can be done to prevent, relieve, and manage pain.

BREAKING THROUGH THE MYTHS

One of the most upsetting aspects about suffering from headache is the truly staggering amount of misinformation circulating about this condition. Friends, coworkers, dentists, optometrists, and psychotherapists may all participate in misdiagnosing and misunderstanding the nature of headache. Not even physicians are exempt. They too may pooh-pooh headache as a minor condition, tell patients that they "just have to live with it," or suggest that the patient's own personality is at the root of the problem.

What a relief, then, to break through the many myths about headache and learn the scientific truth! Let's start by laying out the four principles on which this book is based:

1. Headaches are caused by electrical and biochemical mechanisms in the brain — not by personality, attitudes, or responses to stress. This seems to be true of both migraine and of regularly occurring tension-type headache. (For more on the biology of different types of headache, see Chapter 2.) Although various factors — including stress — can *trigger* this mechanism, a person's predisposition to headache is an inborn, chronic, physical problem. It doesn't "mean" anything about who she is, any more than diabetes, asthma, or arthritis "reveals" anything about the people who suffer from those conditions.

2. There is a wide range of drug treatment that can also help prevent and manage headache. As our understanding of what causes headache expands, so do our medical options. At this point, there are enough treatment options so that a headache specialist or other doctor should be able to find one that works reasonably well for each headache sufferer, with a maximum of effectiveness and a minimum of side effects. (For more about drug treatments for headache, see Chapter 9.)

3. There is a wide range of nondrug treatment that can help prevent headaches from occurring and that can help ease or terminate them when they do occur. Biofeedback, relaxation, visualization, changes in diet, regular aerobic exercise, the use of heat and cold, and a host of home remedies have all been tried by headache sufferers, often with a high degree of success. Psychotherapy and short-term counseling have also proved helpful to some "headache people." (For more about these approaches to headache relief, see Chapters 7 and 8.) And virtually all these techniques can be utilized even if the headache sufferer is also taking medication.

4. Your own attitude — toward yourself, your headaches, and your treatment — can make an enormous difference in preventing and managing headache pain. You didn't choose to be born with a headache-prone condition. You're not *at fault* for it. But you are *responsible* for it — for dealing with your condition in a way that works for you. Although you can't *cure* this condition, you can work with it:

- explore what patterns of diet, exercise, and sleep help keep your head clear
- listen to your body and discover ways to comfort and care for yourself
- take an active role in your relationship with your doctor or other health care provider to develop a plan of treatment— drug, nondrug, or both — that you're happy with

In fact, your willingness to take responsibility — for your body, your behavior, and your treatment — may turn out to be the key factor in getting rid of your headaches!

We've found that one of the cruelest consequences of headache is the sense of being a powerless victim, struck down by a mysterious and uncontrollable event. We're willing to bet that you'll find enormous relief just by shifting your perception from "These headaches happen to me" to "I can anticipate, appropriately respond to, and aggressively treat my headaches."

There's one other way you can take responsibility for treating and managing your headaches. You can learn more about what causes them and how they operate, so that you can listen to your body more intelligently and respond to potential headache triggers more effectively. The right doctor or other health care provider can help you learn more about the particular type or types of headache that have been plaguing you. But for a head start on understanding headache, take a look at Chapter 2.

CHAPTER 2

Understanding Headaches

WHAT IS A HEADACHE?

HOW DOES A HEADACHE HAPPEN, and why does it cause us pain? Understanding how to answer this question for *your* particular headache can be enormously helpful to preventing, managing, and easing your pain. Not only will you have more information about what might be causing your headaches and about what foods, drinks, and situations to avoid, but you will also be able to read your own body more sensitively, zeroing in on the triggers that set off *your* particular headaches.

Pain and the Brain

Despite the unpleasant experience of a headache, the brain itself doesn't feel any pain. The experience of a headache comes from pain that is generated in the face, neck, scalp, and meninges or casing of the brain. It only seems as though this pain is coming from inside your head.

In fact, this illusion is what is known as *referred pain.* You have twelve pairs of cranial nerves that carry information to and from the brain. In addition, you have thirty pairs of spinal nerves that carry information to and from your spinal cord (which in turn is connected to all your major organs). When messages of pain get transferred among these nerves, you may *experience* pain in a different part of the body from where the physical cause of that pain is actually taking place.

For example, when some people have heart attacks, they experience the pain in their arms, rather than around their hearts. And when some people have headaches, although the pain is actually *outside* their heads, they experience it as coming from *inside*. They may also experience it in their jaws (hence migraineurs' frequent appeals to dentists), in their sinuses (hence the common misdiagnosis of migraine as "sinus headache," which is actually not common and which is usually accompanied by a stuffed and runny nose and other cold symptoms), and in their eyes (hence the oft-mistaken attribution of headache to eye problems and the many futile trips to the ophthalmologist).

One pair of nerves, the fifth cranial nerves, carry messages to and from the face, eyes, forehead, sinuses, mouth, teeth, and meninges (the membranes around the brain and spinal cord). Thus, if any one of these areas is affected by a pain-causing event, we may experience the pain as happening somewhere else. A strain on the jaw may "refer" pain to behind the eye. Pain from inflamed and dilated blood vessels in our temples seems to be coming from inside our skull.

Not only does referred pain explain why we sometimes misattribute the source of our pain, but it also points out the brain's role in *interpreting* pain. As it happens, this is a very important aspect of understanding headache.

Pain: Event and Interpretation

When you experience pain anywhere in your body, what happens? The impulses that record the sensation of pain travel from the site of the pain — say, a stubbed toe — into the brain, along one of the cranial or spinal nerves. Your brain then has the job of interpreting this sensation.

The notion of the brain interpreting pain may take some getting used to. We're more accustomed to thinking of pain as an objective event, a direct, unmediated experience of the physical world. In fact, registering awareness of an event—

say, stubbing your toe — is quite separate from feeling *pain* from that event. The physical event of stubbing takes place in the toe. But the ability to feel pain — similar to feeling, say, pleasure, sexual arousal, hunger, thirst, or indifference — takes place in the brain, but only after the nervous system has transmitted the information all the way up from the toe.

Have you ever heard of phantom pain? People who have had limbs amputated report experiencing pain (and other sensations) in their missing limbs, even though there is obviously no physical event to cause the experience. A part of the brain is simply choosing to interpret some electrical or biochemical reaction as "pain" in the missing arm or leg. The limb isn't there — but a person doesn't need a limb to feel the pain; he or she needs only the brain.

This process of interpretation is extremely important, both for understanding your headaches and for understanding how to relieve them. Imagine your brain as a gigantic message center in which huge quantities of information are constantly being routed from place to place. "Transmitters" send these messages; "receptors" receive them. In fact, scientists call some of the brain chemicals that perform these functions *neurotransmitters.*

Although there is still much about brain function that we don't understand, these chemicals seem to play many different and sometimes contradictory roles. The absolute level of these chemicals in our brain — as well as the process of these chemicals' rising or falling — apparently affects how sensitive we are to pain, whether we suffer from depression, how well we sleep, and how we respond to stress.

A major neurotransmitter is known as *serotonin,* which, among other things, regulates our response to stress. (Serotonin is synthesized by our bodies from the amino acid L-tryptophan, found naturally in dairy products, turkey, fruits, and green vegetables; consequently, a diet rich in these substances is often recommended to combat stress.) Serotonin also seems to be involved in the biochemical chain of events that produces headaches, a process that we discuss below.

For the moment, however, let's just stay inside the brain, observing the various chemical reactions that affect our responses to physical events. Serotonin isn't the only neurotransmitter involved. To transmit pain signals, our brain also needs other neurotransmitters such as *dopamine, noradrenaline, substance P,* and *acetylcholine.* Some headache medications operate by affecting the levels of these chemicals in the brain or by blocking these chemicals' effectiveness by altering their receptors. Thus, although the cause of pain is still present, the brain is "protected." Suddenly, the same physical event that once produced a headache is no longer interpreted as pain.

Our body also produces a natural pain reliever: endorphins. Although the brain synthesizes endorphins naturally, they are remarkably similar in structure to the morphine that we produce artificially. And endorphins and morphine affect the brain in similar ways: both somehow interfere with the transmission of messages within the brain in a way that lessens the perception of pain.

Of course, just because a person doesn't feel pain does not mean there's nothing wrong. An exhilarated ballet dancer, absorbed in displaying her dying swan to an adoring audience, may feel only artistic ecstasy while she's before her public — but afterward, backstage, she may discover that she's torn a tendon. The endorphins produced by her physical activity and her emotional state acted just like morphine: they anesthetized her from the pain. Soldiers in battle, athletes on the field, and people in emergencies have been known to have similar delayed reactions.

Our body produces endorphins according to its own rhythms, but we can help it along. Laughing, regular aerobic exercise, and being in love all seem to stimulate the production of endorphins. The more you practice any or all of these activities, the more you're building up your "immunity" to headache. Endorphins don't exactly stop the headache process from happening any more than they cure the dancer's tendon. But they can radically lower your sensitivity to the pain that headaches cause.

On the other hand, taking pain relievers on a regular basis seemingly impairs the body's natural ability to produce endorphins or affects serotonin levels. That's why when you start taking a pain reliever, a low dose may be sufficient — your body's pain-relieving mechanisms are doing the rest of the job. After you've been taking medication for a while, though, your endorphin production may go down, or your serotonergic system may be modified and you need correspondingly more of the synthetic pain reliever.

Endorphins and serotonin don't only insulate us from pain. They also seem to play a role in depression. We believe this is so because lower levels of endorphins and serotonin seem to correlate with depression. You might think, then, that if taking pain relievers lowers endorphin production and decreases the effectiveness of serotonin, it would also cause depression — and in some cases, it seems to. Interestingly enough, many people with frequent migraine also suffer from depression. So raising your natural endorphin production or serotonin levels may benefit your health on many levels.

Muscle and Blood

We've taken a look "inside your head," but what about the outside? After all, even if pain is interpreted inside your head, the physical events that cause pain may take place outside the head. So if you can picture the way your head is constructed, you'll be better able to visualize what's happening to you when you get a headache — or when you're in danger of getting one. And, as explained in Chapters 7 and 8, learning how to "read" your body and your head is one of your major resources in combating headache pain.

Picture two major arteries carrying blood to your face, neck, and scalp. One, the *temporal artery,* runs up from your neck, going below and in front of your ears, passing forward to your upper temple, and from there dividing to run over your scalp.

The other major artery in this region is the *occipital artery.* Along with the temporal, it runs up the back of your head from your neck, but it goes beneath and behind the ears. From there, it divides on each side and runs along the lower back of the skull.

The flow of blood to your face and head is one key element involved in producing headache. Another key element is your muscles:

- The *paraspinal muscles* hold your spinal column, or vertebrae, in place. They run up your spine to the base of your skull, where they and other neck and shoulder muscles overlap. Together, they control your head, neck, and shoulder movements.

- The *temporalis muscles* cover the area over your temples — in front of and above your ear. The temporalis muscles are attached to the lower jaw; tightness in your jaw — clenched teeth — can pass tension on up to these muscles. They, too, are excellent indicators of tension — next time you want a great reading on someone's body language, see whether the person's temples are tightening. To feel your own temples contract, put a finger between the top of your ear and the corner of your eyebrow, and then clench your teeth.

- The *masseter muscle* is a muscle covering the joint made up of the jawbone and the skull (the temperomandibular joint) and is utilized when chewing. Clenching this muscle can generate chronic tension and cause pain. To feel the joint covered by this muscle, put your finger in front of your ear and open your mouth. Then clench your teeth to feel the masseter contract in your cheek.

- The *frontalis muscle* is like a cap covering your forehead and the front of your head. It helps you raise your eyebrows and furrow your brow — and feel your headache. It also interacts with all the small muscles around your eyes, which you need to squint, blink, and open your eyes wider. These interacting muscles can also pass tension back and forth among themselves.

- The *occipitalis muscle* covers the back of your scalp. Although it doesn't move, it does surround the occipital artery and nerve, so tension in this muscle puts pressure on the blood vessel and nerve — a pressure that can bring on headache pain.

- The *trapezius,* or shoulder muscle, is a triangular muscle that covers your shoulder blades and continues on up to your skull. Other head, neck, and shoulder muscles interact with it and with each other. All may be involved in the sensation — and the relief — of headache pain.

Now you have a general picture of what goes on inside and outside the brain. To get a more detailed picture of headache, we now have to consider specific *types* of headache. The two most common are the tension-type headache and the migraine.

TENSION-TYPE HEADACHE

What Is a Tension-Type Headache?

There are actually two types of tension-type headache:
Acute tension-type headaches are specific reactions that may be related to particular emotions or events. Many people get this type of headache after sitting in a cramped position, straining their eyes, getting prolonged exposure to the hot

sun, or dealing with a stressful event in their lives. Such headaches tend not to last more than a few hours and are usually responsive to relaxation, rhythmic exercise, a mild over-the-counter drug, or perhaps a nap. Some 75 to 80 percent of all headaches that people get may be classified as this type — and about 90 percent of the population gets at least one from time to time.

Chronic tension-type headaches, on the other hand, occur more frequently — from four to seven days per week — and last much longer. While acute tension-type headaches come on soon after a stressful event, chronic headaches often appear early in the day, apparently in response to nothing. Some people even wake up with chronic tension-type headaches. Although sleep appears to bring some relief, it's possible that a person who suffers from chronic tension-type headache continually wakes up with a new headache, sometimes daily.

Whereas migraines seem to disable those who get them, tension-type headaches seem more manageable. Although they take an enormous toll on a person's sense of well-being and ability to function at her highest level, they usually allow people to continue with their regular activities. Relaxation seems to help ease these headaches, but ironically the people who get them would often prefer to be active. In some cases, of course, these headaches are so disabling that they require the sufferer to relax or perhaps sleep.

Tension-type headaches usually start in the muscles at the back of the head and neck, working their way up through the forehead. People may have various perceptions of where these headaches begin, but they usually reach both sides of the head, although not always with equal intensity. (Migraines, by contrast, are most often felt on only one side of the head.) Sometimes tension-type headaches progress as far as the temples; sometimes they reach the area just behind the eyes. The sensation has been described as having one's head held in a vise, or having one's head covered in pain as though wearing a tight cap.

In addition to affecting the muscles of the scalp, neck, and forehead, these headaches also seem to bring pain to the shoulders. Sometimes a person with such a headache notices "knots" — tightly tensed muscles — in the neck, shoulders, or back. People who get this type of headache may also experience nausea (although not to the extent that is common with migraine).

People who get such headaches may get them immediately after or during a stressful time, such as while pushing to meet a deadline at work or driving the car in a pouring rainstorm. With migraine, though, the pattern is more subtle: the headache comes *after* the stress has been alleviated, say, on a Saturday morning or on the day after the rainy trip. Frequently, people who get migraine feel that they have to "beat the clock," either at work or at home, and their headaches come only after they feel they have completed their duties.

Another trigger for tension-type headaches seems to be sitting, reading, typing, or driving for long hours in the same position. It's not clear whether the headaches are triggered by the stress of focusing on an activity, by the muscular response to a cramped or fixed position, or by some kind of interaction between the two.

What Causes Tension-Type Headaches?

Actually, both names for this disorder — muscle contraction headache and tension-type headache — are rather misleading. They suggest that such headaches are caused either by contracting muscles or by an overload of tension, and for many years doctors believed this to be true.

Now, however, we think that so-called muscle contraction headaches are more closely related to migraine than had previously been thought and are now called "tension-type headache." This type of headache seems to be caused by the same type of biochemical process that produces migraine; in fact, it may be on a continuum with migraine, so that both are aspects of the same disorder.

In both tension-type and migraine headache, the *serotonergic* system seems to be disturbed. As mentioned earlier, serotonin is the neurotransmitter involved in experiencing pain, regulating sleep, and determining depression. A central system of nerve fibers relies on serotonin and controls the sensation of dull pain, patterns of sleep, emotions, and the sense of well-being. Like migraine, chronic tension-type headache is also often associated with sleep disturbances and depression, which suggests that both types of headache are related to the same type of serotonergic disturbance.

Researchers have hypothesized that some people are born with a biological predisposition that leads them to translate physical and emotional stress into headache: some develop tension-type headaches, others migraine. That many migraine sufferers develop chronic, daily, tension-type headaches in later life suggests that the same central nervous system disorder is responsible for both.

If this hypothesis is true, it seems that the biochemical process not only brings on a headache but may also tighten up a person's muscles in response to pain. Thus, biochemistry, and not tense muscles, may be the ultimate cause behind tension-type headache.

Responding to Tension-Type Headaches

Whether or not these headaches have their source in biochemistry or in tense muscles, one thing is clear: Contracted muscles cause pain. Therefore, learning to relax your muscles can help prevent tension-type headache.

Why is this true? One reason is *ischemic pain*, whereby a part of the body signals that it is experiencing a lack of blood.

If you were to strap a blood pressure cuff tightly around your arm, so that the flow of blood to your forearm was completely cut off, you wouldn't feel any pain in your forearm — until you tried to move it. That's because exercising a muscle under low-oxygen conditions produces increased metabolic waste products. Usually, the free circulation of blood brings high oxygen levels and rinses these products away before they can do any harm. If the blood is not circulating freely, however, the low oxygen supply leads to a buildup of waste products and the nerves are irritated: hence, pain. As soon as you took off that cuff, for example, the pain would subside.

By the same token, if your muscles are tightly contracted — an instinctive response to danger or difficulty — they are interfering with the free flow of blood throughout that part of your body. This overworking of muscles can irritate their contractile fibers and nerves and cause headache pain. And you pay for this contraction for a long time: Only two minutes of tightly contracted muscles can eventually cause pain, which may not disappear until long after the muscles have been relaxed. That's why a person who's been tense and stressed-out all week might wake up relaxed on Saturday morning — with a tension-type headache.

On the other hand, regular aerobic exercise, which helps the blood circulate freely, can be a great antidote to tension-type headaches, restoring circulation and building up your "headache immunity," so to speak. We know one tension-type headache sufferer who made it a point to get at least twenty minutes of aerobic exercise after any stressful day. She found that her "weekend" or "next day" tension-type headaches virtually disappeared.

If you get this type of headache, you don't need to think of yourself as more tense than other people. It's just that your tension translates into a particular biochemical response, which involves tightening your muscles. Just as a diabetic has to be more careful about sugar intake than most people, so might you have to be more careful about muscle tension. Take a look at Chapter 8 for some suggestions on noticing and relieving this type of headache-triggering tension.

Physical Sources of Tension-Type Headache

It may also be the case that your tension-type headaches have a more purely physical source. If you have *arthritis,* for example (an inflammation of the joints), the muscles around your source of pain may instinctively be contracting. Apparently, this is a vestige of the body's "splinting" behavior, in which muscles contract around a broken bone in order to help it heal. Of course, contracting muscles around arthritis pain cause even more pain — and if the arthritis is in your neck, the pain may become a headache.

If the arthritis or another degenerative condition has led to the deterioration of a bone or spinal disc (the cartilage that cushions each of your vertebrae), these structures may compress one of the nerves leaving your spinal cord. Now you've got a *pinched nerve,* which, as it is not fully functioning, may lead to pain, tingling, numbness, or weakness in the area that it serves. A pinched upper cervical nerve may refer pain and tingling up into your head, neck, shoulder, upper back, arm, or hand.

Any other *neck problems* — such as those caused by whiplash, a spinal tumor, or congenital (present from birth) deformities — may also result in tension-type headache. That's because even a slight contracting of the muscles sets up a vicious cycle: the contraction puts pressure on a nerve, causing pain, causing further contraction, causing more pain.

MIGRAINE

What Is a Migraine?

Although the more dramatic forms of migraine may be the most well-known, the severity of migraine headaches range from mild to intense. In fact, the same person may suffer from both mild and severe migraines, sometimes alternating frequently between one and the other, sometimes going through long periods where only one type of headache is experienced. That's why it is so important to be careful in diagnosing migraine, because it isn't reducible to any one collection of symptoms or signs, although it is a fairly recognizable disorder.

According to a strict, technical definition, migraines are throbbing headaches that are felt on only one side of the head. (The word "migraine" is from the Greek *hemikrania*, meaning half the head.) Most migraineurs experience nausea and sometimes vomiting, as well as sensitivity to both light and sound. The pain is worsened by activity (mild exercise or bending over).

Most people who get migraines have at least one by adolescence, although it is possible for migraine to start at any time in your life. Many women migraineurs notice that their migraines start sometime in the months or years after they start menstruating. Some women notice a marked falling-off of migraine during pregnancy, with the headaches coming back after delivery. However, other women get their first headaches during pregnancy or, more commonly, after their first childbirth. Some women notice a definite improvement in their migraines after menopause, while other women get their first such headaches after they've stopped menstruating. Migraine in women seems to correlate somehow with estrogen levels, but the correlations are complicated and vary a great deal from person to person. Generally, falling estrogen levels just before menses are a particularly strong migraine trigger. (For more on menstrual migraine, migraine during pregnancy, and migraine and menopause, see Chapters 4, 5, and 6.)

Some people experience *auras* or sensory disturbances at the beginning of a headache. These attacks are known as *classical migraine* (migraine with aura), the kind of headache suffered by 10 to 15 percent of all migraineurs. A visual aura might include brightly colored, blinking lines; flashes of light;

differently colored dots; black spots; or actual hallucinations. It also might cause a person to see only half an object. Auras may also involve distortions in the other four senses, a feeling of tingling or numbness, trouble with speech, or a general sense of disorientation. Generally, headaches come swiftly on the heels of the aura, within ten to thirty minutes.

The other 85 to 90 percent of migraineurs suffer from *common migraines* (or migraine without aura), which have no dramatic auras, although there may be some warning signs, such as a hot sensation in the head, a feeling of heaviness, or a tightening sensation throughout the scalp. In some people, headache warnings appear many hours or up to one day before the actual attack. These may include changes in mood, energy, and appetite and are called a *prodrome.* Other people experience their headaches with no warning symptoms at all. Still others have never related their warning symptoms to their headaches or ignore the symptoms when they come. Learning to read your own body's warnings and symptoms may be an important part of developing an effective treatment for your headaches.

The migraine itself lasts from four to seventy-two hours, bringing dull, aching pain at first and then overwhelming, throbbing pain; or fluctuating states of pain. Most migraineurs are extremely sensitive to light and noise while they are having their headaches. Moving, bending over, or suddenly changing position may make the headache feel worse. Some migraineurs must lie down; others must remain upright or with their heads at a particular angle; some become dizzy during their headaches. Generally, most migraineurs feel nauseated and sometimes vomit; they may also experience diarrhea, increased urination, and the feeling of anorexia or not wanting to eat.

Most migraineurs feel cold while their headaches are at their worst, particularly in their hands and feet, which are cold to the touch. Just before their migraines, their heads may have felt hot. Formerly, doctors believed these temperature changes were caused by changes in circulation; we now believe that they also have to do with disturbances in a structure deep in the brain called the hypothalamus, our body's "thermostat."

Many migraineurs report being awakened from a deep sleep with a beginning or full-blown headache. Frequently, people get migraines after a period of intense stress has ended, such as on vacation, a weekend, or the day after meeting a deadline.

Other possible neurologic symptoms include aphasia, or difficulty expressing oneself in speech; a tingling or numbness in the lips, tongue, face, or fingers; weakness on one side of the body; double vision; problems with coordination; difficulty thinking clearly; and even amnesia.

After the headache is over, the migraineur may feel drained and washed out, or energized and hungry. Some migraineurs report feeling exhausted for days after their attacks; others experience a new surge of energy and release, as though they are renewed and purged of the tension felt before and during the headache.

What Causes a Migraine?

For years doctors referred to migraines as *vascular headaches,* that is, headaches involving the blood vessels and circulatory system. They used to believe that problems with circulation — perhaps brought on by stress — were the root cause of this disorder.

Now, we believe that an electrical and biochemical dysfunction affecting the brain is the ultimate generator of migraine headaches. However, problems with the circulatory system are certainly involved.

Older theories suggested that migraines begin with *vasoconstriction,* the narrowing of blood vessels either in the brain or carrying blood to the brain. If you've ever felt the jolt of drinking a cup of strong coffee, you know what vasoconstriction is: your blood vessels tighten up, pushing the blood more quickly through your system. However, a more extreme degree of vasoconstriction can actually decrease blood to an area of the brain. Thus, classical migraineurs experience visual disturbances prior to headache; parts of their brains may not be getting the necessary blood.

Although there is a decreased blood flow in the brain, it is caused by a biochemical change. There is also release of certain peptides or chemical messengers (such as substance P) from nerve terminals that irritate the nerves and adjacent blood vessels, causing inflammation in the meninges, or covering of the brain. Unusually high levels of neurokinin A, a substance resembling a component of wasp venom, has been found during a migraine, as has CGRP (calcitonin gene-related peptide) and VIP (vasoactive intestinal polypeptide).

Every action produces a reaction, and vasoconstriction cannot continue forever. It produces its opposite, *vasodilation,* the unusual expansion of blood vessels to include extra amounts of blood. This is one part of the migraine process that we experience as pain: the too-full blood vessels throbbing and pounding along our neck and scalp and on the brain's surface, their nerves inflamed and irritated.

Many hypotheses have been advanced as to what activates this migraine process in the brain. Some scientists believe that the syndrome is triggered by changing levels of sugar and insulin in the blood; missing a meal or eating too-sweet food may thus cause headaches. (For more detail on this theory, see Chapter 7.)

A theory that we find more convincing is that low levels of cerebral magnesium followed by electrical changes in the back of the brain set off changing levels of serotonin. Since the level of serotonin is unusually high before a migraine and unusually low during the headache, we might speculate that this fluctuation sets the vascular problems in motion. The sense of well-being that some migraineurs feel would then be attributable to restored levels of serotonin after the migraine is over. We also know that serotonin constricts blood vessels and that a drop in the serotonin level corresponds to a feeling of depression, which many migraineurs experience just before their migraines begin. The fact that many migraineurs have a family history of depression, as well as one of migraine, gives further weight to this theory and strongly suggests that the tendency to both migraine and depression are inherited together.

A third hypothesis, compatible with the other two, points to *vasoactive substances* — substances that have a definite impact on circulation and vascular activity. We've already mentioned the power of caffeine. You may also have noticed that sometimes taking a cup of coffee or two at the beginning of a migraine can prevent or abort a headache; the coffee acts to constrict the blood vessels, thereby preventing the dilation that brings on headache pain. On the other hand, becoming addicted to coffee can also provoke headaches, since the body starts to depend on the coffee to keep the blood vessels constricted. Without the caffeine, blood vessels may react by dilating, producing a throbbing headache. (For more on diet and headache, see Chapter 7.)

Other foods, medications, and environmental factors may have a similar impact. Learning to read your own reactions to various foods, drugs, and states of weather can therefore be an important aid in treating your migraines.

A fourth hypothesis holds that there is an inflammation in the meninges caused by a release of substance P at the end of the nerves. This causes pain and dilated blood vessels.

There's an interesting link between the serotonin and the substance P theories: serotonin is a nitrogen-containing substance called an *amine*. And many foods that seem to trigger migraine also contain amines, all of which affect the blood vessels, sleep patterns, and a person's mood. (For more on the relationship between amines and migraine, see Chapter 7.)

One theory suggests that the *levels* of amines in the migraineur's system may be the cause of the headache.

Another holds that migraineurs' blood vessels are simply more sensitive to serotonin than the vessels of other people. Thus, migraineurs may simply be more sensitive to *tyramine*, an amine found in such foods as cheese and red wine, and to *adrenaline*, the substance our body produces during periods of stress, and one of a group of chemicals known as *catecholamines*.

Ironically, the body produces adrenaline to mobilize its resources against a possible threat. But the migraineur who reacts to adrenaline by developing a headache may feel that the "protection" is far more painful than any threat could ever be!

MIGRAINE TRIGGERS

As we indicated above, migraines are ultimately *caused* by an inborn biochemical disorder that affects the central nervous system. A person without this disorder can be exposed to a variety of foods, weather conditions, and emotional stressors without ever getting a migraine. A person with this disorder, on the other hand, may be susceptible to a range of migraine *triggers*, physical or emotional factors that set in motion the biochemical malfunction. Thus, even though the triggers don't cause the headache, they may provoke it. Learning which triggers are likely to affect you, and under what circumstances, is one of the best ways to begin your migraine treatment.

Becoming a "migraine detective" and figuring out your "usual suspects" can be a tricky business because a trigger that provokes a headache on one occasion may not do so on another. Some migraineurs notice that if they are relaxed, happy, and generally keeping to a low-sugar diet, they can afford to take a glass or two of white wine. If they are stressed-out or have been eating lots of sweets lately, the same white wine may set off a pounding headache. Likewise, some women have to be especially careful during the days just before, during, or just after their periods, whereas they feel much more "immune" from headaches during the rest of the month.

The headache triggers we identify in this section, then, affect migraineurs in a variety of ways. You may find it useful to make your own list of headache triggers, noting the circumstances under which each is dangerous for you, as well as the conditions, if any, under which the substance or experience may be safe. You may also find it helpful to keep a headache diary of the sort that we recommend on pages 74–75 in Chapter 3.

Weather

Some people who are prone to headache notice that they are more vulnerable during certain kinds of weather: damp, cloudy days; dry, windy days; or days when the barometric pressure is changing in either direction. Some people are also susceptible to the so-called ill winds such as the southern California Santa Ana and the Arizona desert's hot, dry winds. This is probably because winds are generated by changing weather fronts.

Studies of nonmigraineurs' reaction to the Israeli *sharav* and the Balkan bora (cold, rainy weather) showed that, in fact, weather does affect people's biochemistry, via the presence of electrically charged ions in the air. Somehow, when the ratio of charged to uncharged particles changes, the human biochemical system reacts — and in migraineurs, the reaction is often a headache.

Temperature, Humidity, and Pressure

Migraineurs who are sensitive to the weather may also find their headaches triggered by air-conditioning, or the lack thereof, and by shifts in atmospheric pressure, such as those experienced while riding in an airplane. Low-pressure weather fronts, which may bring storms with them, often bring "headache weather" as well; likewise, a cold winter is often a rocky time for "migraine people."

It's also possible that a headache triggered by some other source may be eased or worsened by these atmospheric conditions, e.g., a stress-induced migraine may get worse as the migraineur sits in the humid living room, while going to the air-conditioned bedroom tends to ease the pain.

Altitude

Higher altitudes often set off migraines, because less oxygen is available to the brain. When the migraineur's body tries to compensate by dilating the blood vessels (so that more blood can carry more oxygen to the brain), a throbbing headache may well result. In some cases, people who go as high as eight thousand to twelve thousand feet find themselves with acute mountain sickness, which includes severe headache, vomiting, confusion, lassitude, shortness of breath, and insomnia.

Doctors recommend responding to this condition by descending to an altitude at least three thousand feet lower, inhaling pure oxygen, or taking Diamox or steroids. Some doctors believe that vitamin C may be a helpful nondrug treatment, as it helps the circulation of oxygen throughout the body. Likewise, aerobic exercise prior to going to high altitudes will condition the body so that it will be better able to tolerate high altitudes.

Light

Bright or flickering light seems to set off headaches in approximately 30 percent of all migraineurs. Intense sunlight, strobe lights, or sometimes even faulty fluorescent lights can frequently trigger migraines. A broad-rimmed hat and sunglasses might offer some protection against these migraine triggers when you're outdoors.

Motion

The motion of traveling on a bus, boat, car, or train may set off a migraine in adults, just as it triggers motion sickness in many children who later develop migraine. We don't completely understand why this should be so.

Sleep Changes

Many migraineurs notice that suddenly getting a lot less or a lot more sleep triggers a migraine. Others even more sensitive are headache-prone if their sleep/wake schedule changes at all, say when they go to bed three hours later than normal after a special party or when they cross through several time zones by plane and develop jet-lag headaches.

Migraineurs who notice that sleep changes trigger their migraines should try to keep their sleep habits as regular as possible — even on the weekends! After all, which would you rather have — the pleasure of "sleeping in" or the relief of being headache-free? Other preventive measures may include aerobic exercise, relaxation techniques practiced during the day and before bedtime, and psychotherapy or counseling to deal with significant issues.

The Female Cycle

Many women notice an increased susceptibility to migraine just before, during, or just after their menstrual periods. Others notice either increased or decreased tendency to migraine during other major events in the female cycle: pregnancy, the month after childbirth, and menopause.

These topics are covered in far more detail in Chapters 4, 5, and 6. For now let's just remind you that the time around menstruation is often a sensitive time for female migraineurs. Food, drink, and emotional situations that might leave you headache-free the rest of the month could trigger a migraine during the portion of the month that's most volatile for you. Keeping a headache calendar (as we describe on pages 74–75 of Chapter 3), listening to your body, and knowing that this is an especially sensitive time may all be helpful as you proceed to treat your headaches.

Diet

A whole host of foods, beverages, and medications may trigger migraine. Some of the most common triggers include excessive caffeine (found in coffee, tea, cola drinks, chocolate, and over-the-counter headache medications); nicotine (in both primary and secondhand smoke); alcohol (particularly hard liquor and red wine); cheese and dairy products; Nutra-Sweet and MSG; and foods containing a high amount of processed sugar (especially when eaten on an empty stomach). For more about diet and migraine, see Chapter 7.

Emotional Triggers

As noted above, adrenaline may be involved with migraine. Since the body produces adrenaline whenever it feels the need for "fight or flight" — that is, during all stressful situations — stress or its cessation may contribute to setting off a migraine. Likewise, depression, frustration, anger (particularly suppressed anger), and letdown may be associated with migraine.

Do you have the feeling that emotional triggers are sparking your migraines? If so, we urge you not to use this perception as a source of guilt or self-blame. Remember, migraineurs as a group have no more difficulty handling their emotions than any other type of person. It's just your unfortunate lot to sometimes translate your difficulties into headache, rather than into some other channel. Learning relaxation techniques, exploring your feelings in psychotherapy, or diffusing your stress through vigorous exercise can help interrupt this process, the way insulin interrupts a diabetic's difficulties with metabolizing sugar. You wouldn't view a diabetic as "weak" or "troubled" because he or she needs regular doses of insulin; give yourself the same leeway to need — and receive — whatever will ease *your* condition. (For more about emotional triggers and a range of nondrug responses to migraine, see Chapter 8.)

Travel

Several factors might set off migraines during a trip: changes in sleep patterns, the stress of meeting travel schedules, and the many migraine triggers lurking aboard an airplane (breathing poor-quality air; experiencing changes in atmospheric pressure; sitting in one position too long; drinking alcohol; and eating foods high in salt, MSG, and preservatives).

What can help make your travel headache-free? Allow plenty of time to get to the airport and get seated in your plane; drink at least eight to twelve ounces of water every two hours; avoid alcohol and high-salt foods such as peanuts; walk around the plane for a few minutes every hour or so; and eat lightly on board. If you take preventive headache medication, be sure to do so well before getting on the plane.

Holidays

A combination of emotional and physical factors make holidays a treacherous time for headache sufferers. We've noticed that we get three times our usual number of emergency calls over three-day weekends — and throughout the entire month of December! Alcohol, missed meals, high-sugar, high-salt foods, and other trigger foods like hot dogs and paté, changes in sleeping habits, and the myriad of social and emotional pressures are all potential headache triggers even by themselves, so you can imagine how they reinforce one another in combination.

We'd never suggest missing out on the holiday fun. But to

keep your fun as painless as possible, go easy on the alcohol (especially red wine) and drink twelve ounces of water for every hour you are drinking. (Alcohol inhibits the secretion of the hormone ADH [antidiuretic hormone] from the pituitary gland, causing you to urinate more often and to become dehydrated. This dries out brain cells, lowers spinal fluid pressure, and produces headache. All this is prevented by drinking a lot of water.) Keep high-sugar and high-salt foods to a minimum. Eat foods high in fructose, such as grapes, tomatoes, and honey. Do what you can to keep your sleep as regular as possible. If you are taking pain medication, don't overmedicate yourself: You could be setting yourself up for "rebound headaches," in which your body needs ever-higher doses of the drug. And last but not least, provide yourself with plenty of "support people" to process the stresses with family and significant others that these times seem to inspire in all of us!

MIXED HEADACHES

For many years doctors believed that most headaches fell neatly into two separate categories: migraine and tension-type headache. Recently, however, we have begun to realize that these two disorders may represent two clinical presentations of the same problem. Further evidence for their connection or a continuum of headaches lies in the high-frequency of tension-type headache in migraineurs: the so-called mixed headache syndrome.

Mixed headaches are actually combinations of migraine and tension-type headache. These combinations may appear in various patterns.

When Migraineurs Suffer from Tension-Type Headache

Sometimes a migraineur will unconsciously brace herself against the pain of an incipient or full-blown headache.

Tightening and lifting the shoulders seems to be an instinctive reaction to danger, perhaps stemming from a primitive desire to use the shoulders to protect the head. Although the response is instinctive, it's actually counterproductive, since tightening your muscles only increases the headache pain. Learning relaxation techniques or receiving biofeedback training may help migraineurs who suffer from this type of mixed headache.

When Tension-Type Headaches Include Migraine Symptoms

Sometimes a person whose headaches are basically classified as tension-type headache also suffers from occasional migraine symptoms: digestive problems, nausea, vomiting, sensitivity to light, and other symptoms related to cerebral processes of migraine. Such a person would usually be able to keep working through her headaches — but not always. She might sometimes notice increased pain when her head is held at a certain angle — but not always. Usually, although such a person might wake up with a headache, she is unlikely to be awakened by one.

Vigorous, regular aerobic exercise, careful attention to diet and sleep patterns, and care to avoid an overreliance on pain medication — even over-the-counter drugs — can be very helpful to people with this sort of headache. If you think you have this type of headache and you're seeking medical treatment, make sure your health care provider is familiar with this kind of headache and the concept of analgesic rebound headache, rather than trying to treat you for only one type of headache or the other.

Chronic Daily Headache

Some migraineurs suffer from this headache pattern, in which the migraines "evolve" to include virtually constant dull headaches punctuated by occasional intense migraines.

Also known as *evolutive* or *transformed migraine,* this syndrome is usually developed in a person's thirties or forties, although sometimes it takes place after menopause.

A study of 515 patients with this syndrome found that there was a high correlation with alcoholism, substance abuse, and depression. The study also found that 77 percent of the patients were taking pain relievers every day, a practice that may have been causing "rebound headaches." (In a rebound headache, the body becomes so dependent on the pain relievers that it starts getting headaches as the pain medication wears off several times each day.)

We believe that, once again, the serotonin and/or amine systems are involved in this biochemical disorder. Perhaps the brains of people with chronic daily headache are simply not producing enough serotonin or endorphins, the body's natural insulations against pain. This underproduction may be intensified by the overuse of pain medication, which, as discussed above, tends to lower the body's natural production of pain-relieving chemicals. It's also possible that the brain stem or the hypothalamus is involved in the disorder.

Medicating chronic daily headache is tricky and often involves a period of helping the patient withdraw from pain relievers. However, scientific understanding of this condition is growing all the time. (For more on medical responses to chronic daily headache, see Chapter 9.) As with other types of headache, a range of nondrug treatment may prove remarkably helpful, no matter what the condition's underlying biology.

OTHER TYPES OF HEADACHES

Cluster Headaches

These headaches affect less than one percent of the population, and of those affected, most are men, by a ratio of five to one. Because cluster headaches produce a runny or stuffed nostril and a red and tearing eye all on the same side of the head on which you feel the pain, they are often misdiagnosed as sinus- or allergy-related. In truth they, like migraines, seem to be set off by the constriction and dilation of blood vessels of the head.

Cluster headaches are probably the most painful type of headache there is. Mercifully, they last only thirty to ninety minutes; but while they continue, the pain is remarkably intense and has been described as though a hot poker is thrust into the eye and twirled. Other symptoms include a drooping eyelid and a small pupil.

Some 80 to 90 percent of cluster sufferers have *episodic cluster headache,* in which they get from one to three headaches a day for four to six weeks. Then the person is likely to be headache-free for five months to a year, until the cycle begins again. *Subchronic cluster headaches* are similar, except that the remission lasts less than six months. *Chronic cluster headaches* appear from three times a day to several times a week throughout the year, without remission. Only 10 percent of cluster patients have the chronic form.

Chronic Paroxysmal Hemicrania (CPH)

Women are more likely than men to suffer from this rare form of headache, which is apparently a variant of cluster. The person with CPH gets about fifteen brief headache attacks within twenty-four hours, each attack lasting ten to twenty minutes. Those suffering from CPH will be glad to know that their headache type is extremely responsive to indomethacin (Indocin), an anti-inflammatory medication.

TMJ Syndrome

If your mouth and jaw feel tender while your head aches, you may be suffering from TMJ syndrome: problems with the temporomandibular joint. That joint is where your mandible (lower jaw) attaches to your temporal bone (skull bone). Put your finger in front of your ear and move your mouth — that's your TMJ.

The TMJ syndrome seems to come from a misalignment of the teeth and jaw, which causes the jaw muscles to overcompensate as they try to "push" the jaw into a correct position. Stress, tension, clenching your jaw, grinding your teeth, eating, and talking may all aggravate the area. Frequently, people tense this area or grind their teeth in their sleep.

Dentists may attribute to TMJ syndrome headaches that are actually caused by migraine or some other factors. The pain in the jaw may be only referred pain, rather than the source of the problem. So if someone tells you that your headaches are caused by TMJ syndrome, you might want to get a second opinion, possibly from a TMJ specialist.

How can you tell if your headaches are caused by TMJ syndrome? If you have trouble opening your mouth, or if you hear popping or cracking noises associated with pain while you chew, TMJ syndrome may be at fault. Treatment might include a combination of medical and dental approaches, including a splint or appliance for your jaw to open your bite and biofeedback to help you relax your jaw.

Eyestrain Headaches

As with TMJ syndrome, headaches that appear to be caused by eyestrain may only be referred pain to the eye area. Sometimes, though, frequent squinting to see better does put a strain on the muscles around your eyes, and this strain translates into muscle contraction across your entire head. A trip to the optometrist or ophthalmologist might ensure that your prescription is up to date — or that you have the corrective lenses that you need! — and that you are not allergic to anything in your contact lens–care chemicals.

Sex Headaches (orgasmic)

Some people experience sudden, intense headaches at the moment of orgasm. These are called *benign orgasmic cephalgia,* or sex headaches, and, while not life-threatening, are certainly troublesome. Migraineurs seem more susceptible to this disorder, but other people get it too. Researchers believe that it may be related to the muscle contraction around the neck and shoulders during intercourse, as well as to the central nervous system disorder suffered by migraineurs and dilation of blood vessels in the head.

If your headaches fit this pattern, you should check with your health care practitioner to make sure that nothing more serious is wrong, because in a very few cases, such headaches may indicate an aneurysm, hemorrhaging, or other life-threatening conditions. You may also want to consider whether there is a psychological dimension to your headaches. (For more suggestions on psychological aspects of headache, see Chapter 8.) However, given the muscular and vascular activity during sexual excitement, it's perfectly possible that sex headaches are purely physical in origin. Headache onset prior to sex may signal psychological issues. Headaches during sex are more likely a variant of migraine or organic and caused by another problem.

Ice Pick Headaches

If your headaches feel like brief, piercing jabs and jolts that seem to penetrate various parts of your head, you are probably suffering from this migraine variant. So-called ice pick headaches may occur frequently or only once in a while, with attacks lasting anywhere from a few seconds to several minutes.

Ice pick headaches generally go into spontaneous remission for unspecified lengths of time. However, doctors can treat them successfully with indomethacin.

Benign Exertional Headache

Mild exertion — coughing, sneezing, stooping, bending, or straining in any way — is enough to bring on this type of headache. It's called "benign" because it's not life-threatening, but it may cause you anywhere from several seconds to several hours of intense pain. It too is a migraine variant, and it is often treated with indomethacin.

"B.A.D." HEADACHES: A FEMALE PROBLEM

Although most exclusively female headaches are related to hormonal fluctuations (see Chapter 4), one is not. The "B.A.D." headache — resulting from a "benign autonomic dysfunction" — affects mostly women, but it comes from a benign (non-life-threatening) heart defect.

This defect, known as the *mitral valve prolapse,* involves one of the doors (valves) to a heart chamber not completely closing. This condition may bring on headaches accompanied by chest pain, rapid heartbeat, changes in blood pressure, and possibly some emotional disturbances.

Women who suffer from this type of headache may flush or break out in red blotches on their chests and necks when they are excited, irritated, or under stress. Their pupils may also be unusually large.

Despite the ominous-sounding reference to the heart, this condition is not linked to heart disease, nor does it pose any real danger of any kind. Consequently, it has received very little attention from doctors or the public, although as many as 10 percent of all women may have it — a total of 14 to 15 million women in the United States alone. Female migraineurs are particularly prone to this condition, and some 15 to 20 percent of them suffer from "B.A.D." headaches.

Drug-free treatments for this condition are essentially the same as for most headaches: exercise, a diet low in caffeine and alcohol, relaxation exercises, and an understanding of your body and emotions. Medications that may treat the condition effectively include propranolol HCl (Inderal) or some other beta-blocker.

CHECK IT OUT: WHEN A HEADACHE MEANS DANGER

Some 95 percent of the time, headaches are a *primary* disorder — an illness, not a symptom of a medical problem. In other words, the headache *is* the problem.

The other 5 percent of time, a headache is a *secondary* disorder — the symptom of something else that has gone wrong. That's why, if you suffer from regular headaches, it's vital that you check out your condition with a doctor, to make sure that your headaches aren't signaling the presence of any other disease. It's also important to check out any headache that seems unusual in any way, or outside of your regular headache pattern.

In the unlikely event that your headaches are the symptoms of other types of illnesses, what might they be?

Posttraumatic headache or head injury headache A headache may be your body's response to an injury to the head or neck. Such a headache may develop months or even up to one year after the initial injury. The head pain may signal a subdural hematoma, or blood clot, pressing on the brain; or it may not signify any danger at all. If you can relate a headache to a head injury, or if you start getting headaches that feel different from your usual head pain, be sure to see a doctor.

If you think you're suffering from a posttraumatic injury, you should avoid any pain relievers stronger than Tylenol, as they may cover up important symptoms. Avoid aspirin and other anti-inflammatory medication, such as ibuprofen (Nuprin, Advil), as they may increase your tendency to bleed.

Make sure someone stays with you for the first day or so after the injury and have him or her wake you up every few hours during the first night to see if you can be alert and functioning. Be sure to stay in close touch with your doctor for the first few days.

Temporal arteritis headache After the age of fifty-five, a person may be susceptible to this type of headache, which is caused by the inflammation of an artery in the scalp, usually the temporal artery (which runs through the temples). Generally, this type of headache goes with aches and pains in the body or the limbs, weakness, and with disturbances of vision. If this condition isn't treated promptly, it may lead to blindness or a stroke.

Meningitis headache Meningitis is an inflammation of the meninges, the membranes that surround the brain and spinal cord. It's caused by infection from bacteria or a virus. In addition to intense head pain and a stiff neck, a meningitis headache is associated with nausea, vomiting, fever, and severe weakness. It requires the immediate attention of a doctor and is potentially serious.

Aneurysm headache An aneurysm is a swelling of a blood vessel whose rupture or slow leak causes hemorrhaging into the head. This type of headache brings with it intense pain and often a stiff neck and vomiting. Frequently it also brings mental confusion, lethargy, loss of consciousness, loss of feeling or strength in one or more limbs, or other signs of a stroke. It requires emergency attention.

Brain tumor headache Ironically, this may be the one thing you *don't* have to worry about! People who are seeking help for headache turn out to have brain tumors less than one percent of the time.

Brain tumors do cause headaches — they begin intermittently and progressively gradually grow in frequency and intensity. Usually, though, a headache is one of the last symptoms of a brain tumor. Before the tumor gets to the headache stage, a person is likely to suffer from slurred speech, disturbances of vision or of the other senses, a loss of motor control, personality changes, or seizures.

Warning Signs

Below is a list of warning signs of times when headaches may possibly be signaling something more serious. If you or someone you know is experiencing any of these symptoms with a headache, get to the emergency room immediately:

- fainting
- seizures
- fever of 101 degrees or higher after an injury (a possible sign of brain damage or infection)
- clear fluid or blood coming from the ears or nose (a possible sign of skull fracture)
- lethargy after head trauma
- stiff neck with fever, nausea, and vomiting
- speech problems
- coordination problems
- visual problems
- weakness or numbness on one side

CHAPTER 3

Women and Doctors

I DEALLY, a woman who suffers from headache could rely upon her physician to diagnose her condition properly and to prescribe appropriate treatment. In the best of all possible worlds, a woman's doctor would always treat her with concern and respect; have a thoroughgoing knowledge of the latest research about her condition; and take the time to explore with her the ways that diet, exercise, and emotional issues may be affecting her as well.

Unfortunately, we don't live in that optimal world. Some 59 percent of women with migraines have not been diagnosed by a physician. When women do go to a doctor, headache is frequently misdiagnosed. Many doctors, dedicated and respectful though they may be, are simply not familiar with the vast literature that has developed on the diagnosis and treatment of headache. Other doctors, perhaps more knowledgeable, may be less aware of the role played by lifestyle and psychology as well as by biology. And, sad to say, there are still many doctors who simply do not take women seriously, dismissing their complaints of headache pain with a routine prescription for painkillers or tranquilizers.

Both male and female patients' dissatisfaction with their medical evaluation for headache has been documented by a report presented to the 1991 International Headache Congress. According to that survey, of 136 chronic headache patients, only 30 percent were fully satisfied with their treatment. Some 45 percent said the medications prescribed by their doctors just didn't work. One patient in three felt that his or her doctor was poorly informed about headache.

Of course, we have to allow for a certain level of dissatisfaction that any patient might feel with a doctor while a treatment is still being sought. Looking for headache remedies can be a long and arduous process, through no fault of the doctor. Some patients, suffering intensely from painful headaches, understandably wish that their doctors had the godlike power to grant instant relief — and then express vehement disappointment that this is not the case. It's also true that some patients balk at a doctor's suggestions for necessary changes in their lifestyle, diet, exercise habits, or sleep patterns, preferring to blame the doctor for their ignorance.

Nevertheless, the survey indicates a serious level of patient dissatisfaction with their physicians. If patients have felt this frustration with doctors in the past, it may account for why they don't continue to seek out physicians — or other health care providers — for help with their headaches.

The good news, though, is that many doctors *do* possess both a sophisticated scientific knowledge of headache and a holistic and respectful approach to their women patients. It's true, too, that if you raise some of these issues with your doctor — for example, asking about the role of diet or pressing for more information about a medication's possible side effects — you may be able to work more effectively with him or her. Sometimes doctors believe, rightly or wrongly, that their patients want only the short and simple answers. A patient who makes clear that she is ready for more involvement in her own treatment may be favorably surprised by the response she gets.

In this chapter, we offer suggestions on how to get the most out of your relationship with your doctor. First we must analyze some of the problems — some common roadblocks that can come up in the diagnosis and treatment of headache. Then we describe the kind of treatment that we think a woman with headache has a right to expect: a treatment grounded in respect, a holistic approach, and a certain level of medical expertise. The checklist on pages 55–56 helps you determine whether you're getting everything you deserve from your current physician.

We next suggest some ways that patients and doctors can work together more effectively. After all, if doctors have responsibilities in the doctor-patient relationship, patients must have responsibilities as well. Once you decide to become an equal partner in your own treatment, there are a lot of things you can do to help your doctor diagnose your condition and evaluate your treatment. You'll also be in a much better position to give every treatment option the best possible chance for success.

Finally, if you decide that your current physician is not for you, we offer some suggestions on how to seek a health care provider with whom you can work more effectively. Whatever your experience, we urge you not to give up! Help for your headaches *is* available, even if it takes a bit of work to find the help that is right for you.

WHAT MIGHT GO WRONG

Sadly, all too many doctors have a tendency to overmedicate without regard to side effects. This tendency is especially problematic in the treatment of headache, since headaches are often part of a syndrome of related ailments, including high blood pressure, high cholesterol, sleep disturbance, depression, and anxiety. A medication that treats one aspect of the syndrome may actually make another aspect worse, leading to the need for more medication, in turn causing new problems — and so on and so forth, in a vicious cycle that may actually make the patient sicker.

In one extreme example — unlikely, but possible — a woman with migraine might be prescribed ergotamine, a medication commonly used to reverse a migraine headache. However, ergotamine tends to raise a person's blood pressure, so if the woman has a tendency to hypertension — as many women migraine sufferers do — the ergotamine may make it worse. If the doctor were to prescribe a common beta-blocker — say, propranolol HCl (Inderal) — hoping to bring her blood pressure down, the woman might find that the new medication has raised her cholesterol. (High cholesterol is not uncommon in women with high blood pressure.) Yet the anticholesterol diet that is then prescribed may actually aggravate her migraines!

Furthermore, many of these medications tend to lead to weight gain — which, of course, further increases high blood pressure. Now the woman, suffering from headaches *and* weight gain, is feeling depressed and helpless — a mood that may well be heightened by the drugs she is taking. If the doctor's response to her depression is to prescribe tranquilizers, the woman may become more depressed or slightly disoriented and less effective in her decision making, thereby increasing her sense of helplessness and inadequacy, raising her general level of stress, furthering her depression — and triggering more headaches! Medication that was originally intended to treat this woman's migraines has not only brought on a plethora of side effects — increased hypertension, weight gain, depression, and disorientation — but has also made her headaches even worse.

Another common problem in headache treatment is a doctor's focus on symptoms rather than on the problem as a whole. A doctor who sees headache merely as a pain to be killed rather than as the symptom of a larger process is likely to treat headache with painkillers. Such a doctor may not help you understand which side effects you should look out for. He or she may schedule your visits too infrequently, not giving either of you a chance to monitor your progress and perhaps adjust your dosage.

Overprescription of painkillers can also set off the analgesic rebound effect, a syndrome in which painkillers actually end up making headache pain worse and more constant. A person who takes a headache medication — whether aspirin, Tylenol, ibuprofen, or a prescription medication — may at first experience some relief. As she takes more and more painkillers, however, a biological reaction sets in. Gradually, the body becomes used to the painkillers; and as they wear off, the headache returns. A person who takes too many painkillers, or takes them too often, may discover the need to increase continually their dosage and frequency, to combat the headaches that set in as soon as they wear off. An experienced physician is aware of this effect and works to circumvent it; a doctor who is not aware of it may simply up your dosage.

Such a doctor is not likely to help you develop a holistic approach to headache prevention. Rather than working with you to intercept headaches before they start — through a combination of preventive medication, diet, exercise, and stress management and setting limits on pain relievers — this type of doctor simply increases your dependence on medication, perhaps even leading to the creation of new medical problems, as in the example above.

Another problem we've noticed is that doctors dealing with women patients may tend to overprescribe tranquilizers. Even when they aren't dealing with headache patients, doctors seem to have a tendency to overprescribe these medications for women. Thus, Valium, a powerfully addictive tranquilizer, became one of the most overprescribed drugs in the United States, and one of the most abused: because doctors had inappropriately prescribed it for women. Today, many doctors use Ativan and Xanax in a similar fashion. If your doctor thinks that you simply need a pill to help you "calm down," he or she isn't very likely to help you find diet and exercise patterns that combat your headaches, nor to help you discover therapies and relaxation techniques that can help prevent your pain.

We certainly aren't condemning medication — we've used it with many of our patients to good effect. However, any doctor who prescribes medication must take the time to teach his or her patients all about it: how it works, what its side effects might be, when the patient should call the doctor to report a disturbing development. If your doctor has earned your trust by the way he or she prescribes medication, you can be happy you're in good hands. If not, we urge you to look further, either by opening up the conversation with your current physician or by finding another doctor. Effective help doesn't have to include unpleasant side effects!

Finally, we're sorry to say that all too many doctors have a tendency to focus on medication to the exclusion of other issues. Even doctors who are aware of the latest discoveries in headache remedies and are willing to take the time to explore various dosages and combinations may be inclined to ignore a more holistic approach. In some cases, headaches can be helped dramatically by such nondrug treatments as adjusting your intake of caffeine, eating regular meals, getting at least twenty minutes of continuous aerobic exercise several times a week, and cutting out nicotine and alcohol. In other cases, exploration of dietary triggers can yield rich results. In still other cases, becoming aware of your emotional patterns and learning about ways to relax, to assert yourself, or to view yourself differently can make a radical difference in headache frequency and intensity. A wise doctor helps a patient explore herself — her body, her lifestyle, her emotions — so that whether or not medication is prescribed, the patient learns what her headache triggers are and how to avoid them. Yet all too often, both doctor and patient believe that the doctor's responsibility ends with prescribing appropriate medication — important as that may be.

As doctors ourselves, we're certainly not making a wholesale condemnation of the medical profession. We know of many holistic, responsible, and knowledgeable doctors whose pharmacologic treatment of headaches has helped countless patients. Unfortunately, though, doctors who fall into the errors we've described are far more common than they should be.

EVALUATING YOUR CURRENT HEALTH CARE PROVIDER

Let's start with your current treatment relationship. Is it working for you? How should you evaluate your present health care provider? Here are some of the things we think that all patients have a right to expect:

- Are you treated with respect? Does your doctor give you the chance to explain your concerns, both about your headaches and about your treatment? Does your doctor respond adequately to your concerns, or does he or she dismiss, ignore, or belittle them?

- Are you being given enough information? Does your doctor take the time to explain all of a medication's possible effects and side effects, making clear the limits of what the medication can do as well as its benefits?

- Is your doctor getting enough information? Is he or she aware of your history with other medications? Are you assured that he or she is taking your entire medical history into account, particularly with regard to menstrual history, hypertension, cardiovascular or circulatory problems, family history of such problems, weight gain, cholesterol levels, and depression?

- Does your doctor have a holistic approach? Is he or she aware of your diet, exercise, sleep patterns, and general lifestyle demands? If you have a new source of stress — a new job, problems with a child, financial difficulties — is he or she aware of it? Is your doctor encouraging you to use behavioral and holistic as well as drug-related approaches to prevent and manage your headaches? Do you share the same understanding about the role that drugs should play in your treatment? That is, have the two of you agreed that you will remain on medication indefinitely, or is your doctor committed to getting you off medication in the foreseeable future (if possible)?

- Is your doctor available to you? Can you call him or her — or a knowledgeable medical office staff member — between visits, particularly when you become concerned about the possible effects or side effects of a new medication? Can you schedule an appointment quickly, if necessary, with your doctor or another member of his staff? Has your doctor helped you understand when your reactions to a medication might constitute an emergency, when they might warrant a quick appointment, and when they probably only need to be discussed over the phone? Is your doctor available on an emergency basis at night and on weekends?

If some doctors have a tendency to hoard information or to hand down prescriptions in a superior and unapproachable manner, it's equally true that some patients have a tendency to idolize doctors, expecting godlike wisdom and magical cures from practitioners who are, after all, only human. So if your doctor does not seem to be fulfilling all the points on this checklist, we urge you to work with him or her before looking elsewhere. Perhaps your doctor is simply tired and overworked but would nevertheless be responsive to your request for more information or more time to discuss your concerns. Perhaps your doctor has assumed that you, like many people, would be resistant to a holistic approach and so has hesitated to bring it up. Perhaps your assertive request for a more equal partnership of healing will inspire your doctor to treat you with more respect.

Certainly you should bear in mind that the treatment of headache is a complicated and involved procedure. It's quite possible that your doctor, however competent and committed, may not be able to prescribe instantly your "perfect" medication — the one that works effectively, right away, with no upsetting side effects. It's more likely that you and your doctor will have to work together to come up with the right combination of drug and nondrug treatment; with the right dosage and medication schedule; with the right plan for beginning, continuing, and perhaps ending your use of medication. For treatment to be effective, you have to take an active role: noting side effects and reporting them at appropriate times; following the dosage and schedule that's been prescribed; giving the agreed-upon nondrug treatments a reasonable try.

However, your doctor also needs to be receptive to this activity on your part. He or she needs to listen to the discoveries you've made, take seriously your concerns about side effects, and commit either to continuing your treatment until you're satisfied or to referring you to someone else. Some doctors may not want such a partnership with their patients; some may need to be educated into one; and some may respond to the notion very well. Only you can tell whether your current physician is responsive enough to the notion of a treatment partnership to make staying with him or her worthwhile.

BECOMING A PARTNER IN YOUR TREATMENT

We have found a book by Debra L. Roter and Judith A. Hall, *Doctors Talking with Patients/Patients Talking with Doctors: Improving Communications in Medical Visits* (Westport, CT: Auburn House, 1992), very useful in thinking about the doctor-patient relationship. The authors identify four different types of doctor-patient relationships:

1. Paternalism In this all-too-common relationship, the doctor is the "fatherly" source of power and authority — even if the doctor is a woman! The female patient, on the other hand, is expected to behave like the prototypical good daughter: submissive, obedient, unquestioning, perhaps a bit worshipful.

Certainly it can be a relief to turn over the responsibility for your health to an all-knowing medical authority, who in turn promises to use his or her vast wisdom to make you all better. However, we don't believe this is a very productive relationship, for either doctors or patients. Particularly for headache, which can only be diagnosed and understood through the patient's own description of symptoms (neurological and other tests only serve to confirm that nothing *besides* being headache-prone is the problem), a paternalistic relationship is often counterproductive to finding effective treatment.

2. Consumerism In this relationship, the tables are turned. The "doctor-seller" has relatively less power; the "consumer-buyer" has far more. If the consumer doesn't like what the doctor is "selling," she's free to take her business elsewhere, giving the doctor a huge incentive to please his or her "customer."

The problem with this model is that sometimes a doctor's job is to help the patient face unpleasant truths or to say things she may not want to hear. A patient who resists giving up coffee, for example, despite all the persuasive evidence that it may be worsening her headaches, needs to be confronted with the truth that there's something she could do to help herself get better — and she's not doing it. A patient who insists on being prescribed ever-higher doses of painkilling medication may be both risking an addiction and setting herself up for the painful "rebound" headaches that often occur when medication is taken too frequently or in too great a dosage. (For more about "rebound" headaches, see Chapter 9.) A doctor may have the responsibility to confront the first patient and to limit narcotic relief to the second. Yet if doctor and patient both consider that "the customer is always right," the doctor will be unable to fulfill her or his responsibility.

3. *Default* Sometimes neither the doctor nor the patient takes an active responsibility for the treatment. The doctor prescribes medication according to conventional wisdom, and the patient takes it. Neither attempts to explore the lifestyle or emotional patterns that may be triggering the headaches in the first place; neither actively seeks improvement in the prescribed medication, so long as the side effects are more or less manageable and the pain relief more or less acceptable. Whereas the paternalistic relationship gives all power to the doctor and the consumer relationship gives all power to the patient, this third type of relationship ends in default: the treatment doesn't really succeed very well, and neither party takes any responsibility for it.

In a sense, the default relationship is one of defeat. Both the doctor and the patient have tacitly or explicitly bought into the myths that headache is a relatively minor disorder that doesn't warrant serious treatment and that headaches can't really be managed or prevented. In so doing, both doctor and patient are abandoning some very real possibilities for improving the patient's life.

4. *Partnership* Actually, Roter and Hall call this type of relationship "mutuality," but we prefer the term "partnership" — it's more specific. In this relationship, as the name suggests, doctor and patient become partners in treatment. Both have areas of expertise and areas of ignorance. Both have to do a certain amount of exploring and experimenting. Both have a stake in solving the same problem: preventing and managing the patient's headaches. If the partnership is interrupted by differences of opinion, philosophy, or values, the partners agree to share their disagreements with one another, so that both may arrive at a new agreement.

How might this work in practice? Say your doctor tells you that you have to cut out caffeine if you ever hope to beat those weekend migraines. In your opinion, a hot cup of coffee with milk and sugar is the only thing that makes life worth living. You just can't believe that something that makes you feel so good is also making you feel so bad. What will each of you do?

In a paternalistic relationship, you might just have to grin and bear it. The doctor would tell you his or her opinion, you would tacitly seem to agree — and then you would either submit to the decree or secretly resist it and "forget" to tell your doctor about your lapses.

In a consumer relationship, you'd just tell your doctor that you weren't going to give up coffee and demand that he or she find another solution for you. Some doctors might do so, others might let you go in search of a second opinion; but neither, in this type of relationship, would work with you to help you understand the reason for her or his suggestions.

In a relationship of default, your doctor might tell you to cut out caffeine and then never follow up to see if you did. Or the doctor might listen to your complaints and objections, shrug, and say, "I've given you my opinion; now it's up to you."

In a partnership, however, both of you take an active responsibility for finding solutions to your problem. When your doctor presents you with a difficult solution, you don't just object or submit, you discuss. "Gosh, doctor, I can't imagine giving up coffee. First, I'm afraid of the headaches I'd get from withdrawing. Second, I really love my coffee. Isn't there some other solution?"

The doctor then has several choices. He or she might talk with you further, explaining the biochemical consequences of drinking coffee in your condition. Once you understand how the coffee is affecting you, you may be more willing to give it up. He or she might also suggest ways of gradually reducing your caffeine intake that would help you avoid caffeine-withdrawal headaches.

Alternatively, the doctor might also help you work out a plan for cutting back on coffee, rather than eliminating it completely or all at once. Perhaps knowing that you can have one cup of coffee each day would make it possible for you to cut back. Or perhaps agreeing to a caffeine-free period of four weeks would work for you, since you know that you'll get some coffee again soon. You and your doctor may be gambling that once you've seen how much better you feel without coffee, you'll find it easier to keep abstaining.

Or perhaps it really *isn't* necessary for you to give up caffeine, so long as you cut out alcohol and cigarettes. Perhaps you and your doctor can come up with a system of treats that help you rid yourself of coffee; or perhaps you *will* decide to grin and bear it, because at this point you have so much trust in your doctor! In a partnership, the possibilities are endless.

If you have given your current physician a fair shot at developing a partnership and have still been disappointed, don't give up. Read on for some suggestions on how to find a new health care provider who is more responsive to your needs.

LEVELS OF CARE: WHO ARE YOU LOOKING FOR?

Before you can find the health care provider that you need, you have to know whom you're looking for. Below is a brief overview of the types of healers that you might choose from, as well as suggestions on how to tell which type is right for you.

Primary-Care Physician

Another primary-care physician might be the most effective solution to your headache problem. The advantages to finding another general practitioner, family practitioner, internist, or gynecologist are many: of all the medical doctors you might consider, they are most likely to engage in a long-term medical relationship with you; if they're also treating you for other problems, they'll know about a range of medical conditions that might shed light on your headache syndrome; and they may develop relationships with other members of your family, giving them a more holistic perspective on you and your medical history.

The disadvantages, of course, are that doctors at this level are less likely to have the specialized knowledge that you may need. How severe and disabling your headaches currently are, and how urgent you feel about treating them, determine whether you want to take the time to get to know another doctor at this level.

Specialist (Non-neurologist)

It's possible that one of the following types of specialists could help you with headache and related problems: endocrinologist, orthopedist, ophthalmologist, otolaryngologist (ear, nose, and throat doctor), rheumatologist, allergist, dentist, or oral surgeon. Such a specialist would probably help, however, only if you have a condition that mimics migraine, rather than if you actually do suffer from migraine, tension-type headache, or mixed headache. If your headaches are diagnosed by one of these specialists as the symptom of another type of problem, we suggest you get a second opinion.

Neurologist

Usually if your headaches are severe and persistent, your doctor refers you for at least some neurological evaluation. A neurologist is the specialist to determine whether your headaches are caused by some more serious disorder. Most often, however, they are not; and at that point, most neurologists are probably not interested in treating you. (The exception, of course, is a neurologist who specializes in treating headache; see "Headache Specialist" below.) If your headache treatment has not brought you any relief, you may want to consult a neurologist just to make sure that your head pain isn't caused by a more serious problem. If you're sure that they're "just" headaches, you might want to go to a headache specialist.

Headache Specialist

An internist, neurologist, psychiatrist, or psychologist might specialize in the diagnosis and treatment of headache. Such a doctor is most likely to know the best and most cost-effective way of treating you, based on years of experience with patients who have similar problems and based on her or his own abiding interest in your type of ailment. Just be sure you choose a specialist who really has the expertise claimed; there's no credentialing process for headache specialists, so any M.D. or Ph.D. is free to claim specialized knowledge that he or she might not actually have. Be sure, too, that your specialist has the same commitment to a holistic approach as you do, so that the two of you can agree on the role that medication plays in your treatment.

Treatment Program

Some patients find that specialized care is not enough; they need to enter a full- or part-time treatment program as well. A headache center, either freestanding or affiliated with a hospital, is the place to find this type of treatment, which usually offers an integrated range of services, including helping you to withdraw from ineffective opiate pain relievers. Staff at these programs is most often made up of a team of doctors, nurses, psychologists, and other clinicians under the supervision of a headache specialist. Many patients, particularly those who could not be helped in other ways, find that the individualized focus of a treatment program is what they needed to solve their particular headache problems.

You usually have to be referred to such a program by a

doctor, but sometimes you're able to self-refer as well. Be careful about the program you enroll in, however, since many are not accredited. Since there is no system of accreditation, it's often difficult to tell which centers are legitimate and helpful; you might want to ask a doctor you trust for his or her opinion, or contact the American Council for Headache Education (ACHE). (More information on ACHE is available in the following section.) The National Headache Foundation provides similar services as well.

Chronic Pain Treatment Program

Unlike the headache center, a chronic pain treatment program focuses specifically on helping patients manage pain, often in conjunction with withdrawing from ineffective or overused pain medication. By helping people develop alternative ways of managing pain, these programs help to make medication less necessary. These alternative methods are particularly valuable for headache sufferers since, as has been discussed, painkilling medication often ends up bringing on more headache pain as the effects of the medication wear off.

Often the care provided at these programs focuses exclusively on pain management, however. If you need other types of attention for your headache, a chronic pain treatment program may not be your optimal choice. On the other hand, if you are overusing painkillers and if there is no specialized treatment program nearby, this may be your best option. If you can't get your own doctor to refer you (a doctor's referral is almost always necessary), contact the program anyway; it may be able to refer you to a doctor who will in turn refer you.

Alternative Health Care Provider

Many patients have found relief from alternative health care modalities: holistic or natural nutritionists, chiropractors, acupuncturists, and doctors of Chinese medicine. While there is less scientific evidence to support these healers' claims, it is true that people do frequently find them helpful.

A number of people have reported success with a variety of alternative treatments. *Acupuncture,* part of the system of Chinese medicine, involves using tiny needles — the size of a piece of thread — to stimulate various key "energy centers" in the body. Proponents believe that the treatment helps to balance the flow of energy and electricity through the body. Migraineurs who have undergone acupuncture say that the experience is in fact like the feeling they get after a headache passes.

Chiropractic is based on the fact that every one of the body's organs is connected to the spinal cord. Chiropractors believe that when an organ is distressed, the results can be felt in the spinal cord, throwing the back out of alignment; likewise, a problem in the back's alignment affects the corresponding organ. Many people have found that a chiropractor's work on their muscles and organs, by way of the treatment of the spinal cord, helps prevent or in some cases relieve their headache.

Herbalists, nutritionists, naturopaths, and *homeopaths* work with various combinations of vitamins and other natural ingredients to address headache. Often you can find a chiropractor or an acupuncturist who also knows about nutrition and/or herbal medicine.

The best way to find treatment is through a referral because you can at least be sure that others have found the treatment useful and have felt comfortable with the person's ability to fulfill his or her claims. If you don't know anyone who has explored this type of health care, you might check the bulletin board of your local health food store or natural foods restaurant or strike up a conversation with the people who work there. We caution you, though, to make sure that a medical doctor has at least determined that nothing "worse" than headaches is wrong with you before you seek treatment outside the medical community.

CHOOSING THE DOCTOR WHO IS RIGHT FOR YOU

Once you determine the level of health care that you're looking for, how can you find the provider that you need? Finding the right doctor may take a little patience and creativity, but if you come out of it with a physician whom you trust and respect, the effort is worth it in the end. The following are some approaches that may work for you.

Professional Referrals

Possibly your own doctor realizes the limits of her or his specialization in this field and can recommend you to someone more knowledgeable about headache. Likewise, neurologists, dentists, and ophthalmologists you may have seen for various headache-related problems may be able to send you to a specialist whom they trust.

Private Referrals

Put the word out to friends, neighbors, everyone you know. You never know who else may suffer from headache — or who might be related to a headache sufferer. Perhaps a friend, colleague, relative, or neighbor knows someone who feels that a health care provider helped her. It may be worth an introductory visit.

Contact a Headache Organization

The American Association for the Study of Headache (AASH) is the leading professional society of physicians and other health care providers dedicated to researching the causes and treatments of headache. Nearly one thousand physicians belong to this organization, which offers training courses, meets annually, and publishes a journal, *Headache*, ten times a year. Members of AASH have also founded the

American Council for Headache Education (ACHE), a non-profit organization dedicated to improving the lives of people with headache and helping headache sufferers to work directly with AASH members to support education, research, and advocacy. The Headache Consortium of New England (HCNE) and the National Headache Foundation (NHF) are also good resources.

Find a Headache Support Group

The Rocky Mountain Headache Association and the Florida Headache Association are both nonprofit groups helping people with severe, chronic headache get information, education, and support, while educating the public through publications, seminars, support group meetings, and lists of qualified doctors. Committed to founding other regional support groups along these lines, ACHE may have information about incipient activity in your area.

STARTING A RELATIONSHIP WITH A NEW DOCTOR

When patients come to us for headache treatment, they often bring with them the accumulated frustrations of numerous trips to medical, dental, and other professionals. By the time they see us, they have usually heard myriad explanations for the sources of their headaches, along with proposed explicit or implied treatments for them:

"The ear, nose, and throat doctor I saw told me my head pain was from sinus infections."
"The allergist told me it was clearly allergic."
"The nutritionist said it was hypoglycemia."
"The dentist said I had problems with my temperomandibular joint."

"The psychiatrist said I was overcontrolled, perfectionistic, and tense."

Our job at this point is not to promote our own specialties at the expense of our colleagues'. On the contrary, we need to be as open as possible, getting to know the patient and remaining open-minded to the wide variety of possible sources and triggers that may be setting off her headaches. Where a previous specialist may have insisted on seeing the patient through the lens of her or his own specialty, we must stand back and try to get a more holistic view.

We urge you, therefore, to find a doctor or other health care provider who approaches you and your condition with similar openness. And we urge you, too, to approach your doctor in that same open spirit.

Some of the questions that we like to ask our patients during an initial consultation are listed below. If your new doctor or other provider asks similar questions, you can safely surmise that she or he is going to treat you as a whole person, rather than as a set of symptoms. You might also consider sharing the answers to these questions with your doctor or even writing down the answers before you get to the doctor's office. It might help you remember all the important information you want to share — and you may come to some new insight about your headaches on your own!

Questions Your Health Care Provider May Ask

- Why are you coming here for treatment now?
- What has been your experience with previous physicians or other types of treatment?
- What didn't work for you in previous treatments?
- What do you do for a living?
- How are things going at work these days?
- What are your hobbies and interests?
- What's your home and family situation like?

- How have things been going with your friends recently?
- What would be a typical day for you, from the time you get up until the time you go to sleep?
- How do you think your headaches have affected your life: at home, at work, at play?

It's your physician's responsibility to take your history and explore with you the dimensions of your headache experience. But it's your responsibility to evaluate your physician and your own responses to her or him. Here are some questions that you might ask yourself during this initial consultation, to see if this is a doctor with whom you want to enter a partnership:

Questions to Ask Yourself about Your Health Care Provider

- Is this person taking my pain seriously? Or is she or he challenging the reality, intensity, or debilitating effects of my pain?
- As this person asks me about my lifestyle, my relationships, and my emotions, do I sense respect for my condition, or am I hearing, "Your headaches are your own fault"?
- Does this person seem willing to enter into an active partnership with me, as opposed to a relationship of paternalism, consumerism, or default?
- Will this person be willing to admit that a treatment doesn't seem to be effective and work with me to find another?
- Will this person take seriously my concerns about side effects and work with me to find a treatment I can live with?
- Is this person interested in the actual conditions of my life, and will he or she suggest drug or nondrug treatments that are appropriate to my lifestyle and responsibilities?
- Can I expect this person to explain all tests and medications

to me and to share with me the latest theories on my type
of headache?

- Does this person have a positive attitude, believing in me
and in our mutual ability to relieve my headache pain?

In addition to asking yourself *about* your new health care
provider, you may need to ask her or him some questions.
Here are some that you may find useful:

Questions to Ask Your Health Care Provider

- Have you treated many people with my type of headache?
- What do you think causes my type of headache? (If the
person isn't aware of the latest research on biochemical
causes, as outlined in Chapter 2, she or he may not be a
knowledgeable provider.)
- Do you believe that headache treatments work? (Watch
out for the doctor who tells you, "Headache pain is just
something you have to live with.")
- What will you do if you prescribe something that doesn't
work or that causes side effects that I can't live with?
- Can you give me a written plan for my treatment that
includes what medication to take and how often, what to
do in the event of various side effects, and what to ask for
if I have to go to the emergency room?
- Are you interested in exploring nondrug treatments?
Which ones? (Possible options include learning biofeedback and other relaxation techniques, experimenting with
changes in diet, exploring sources of stress and emotional
issues, and finding a doable kind of regular aerobic
exercise.)
- Do you think I'll ever be able to do away with medication
entirely? (If this is an important goal for you, be sure to
share that concern with your provider and see how she or
he reacts.)
- Can you work with me to develop a payment plan that we

both can live with? Is there someone in your office who can help me negotiate my insurance claims?

THE INITIAL CONSULTATION

At our headache center, we spend a good three to four hours taking a history, doing a neurological examination, running tests, explaining our perspective to the patients, and planning a treatment. Our center is a tertiary care facility, meaning that it is the third level of specialized care available to patients. A primary-care doctor or secondary-care neurologist will not spend this amount of time on an initial consultation, but we find it hard to believe that a thorough exploration can be done in far less than one hour.

We also provide patients with a questionnaire to be filled out before the first visit, including information about previous medication (including over-the-counter drugs); medical and surgical history; family medical history; and dietary patterns, especially with regard to caffeine and alcohol (two major headache triggers!). If your doctor has not provided you with a questionnaire, again, you may want to write down this information to have it available at your initial consultation.

Be especially careful about recording what medication you have taken, in what dosages, and on what schedule. We've frequently seen patients whose medication has not worked for them because of inappropriate dosage amounts, poor timing of dosing, or failure to follow instructions. We've also seen all too many patients who, while taking prescribed medication to *prevent* their headaches, were never encouraged by their doctors to stop taking prescription or over-the-counter medication intended to *relieve* their headaches. These pain relievers often interfere with the efficacy of other medication, dooming the treatment to failure before it starts!

Taking a History

A major part of our initial consultation is taking a patient's headache history. Our method for doing so is outlined below, so that you may prepare for a possibly similar approach from your own doctor.

We begin by asking patients to rate their headaches on a scale of one to three. A level three headache is *severe,* leaving the patient totally incapacitated. A level two headache is *moderate;* while painful and clearly a problem, it allows the patient to continue to function — although it may interfere with optimal performance. A level one headache is *dull;* this relatively mild pain does not interfere with the patient's functioning and may even go unnoticed while the patient's attention is absorbed elsewhere.

Then we explore other characteristics of each type of headache. For each level of intensity, we ask the following questions:

- How old were you when you first started getting this type of headache? What were the circumstances?
- How often do you currently get this type of headache? Has this changed over the course of your life? When did it change? Do you have any sense of why — change in lifestyle, new treatment, cessation of treatment, etc.?
- Where do you experience this headache: in your forehead? Top of head? Back of head? Temples?
- Does this pain feel more intense on the right or the left side? Do you feel it on both sides? Does it alternate sides? If you have both right- and left-sided headaches, does one side predominate?
- Describe the pain: Is it throbbing, pounding, pulsating, squeezing, pressing, aching? (Most patients can accurately describe their own pain, but for those who can't, we give them a list of descriptive words to choose from.)

- How long does this type of headache usually last? What's the longest it has ever lasted? What's the shortest?
- What happens to you before you get the headache? Do you notice any changes in appetite, energy, mood, sleep patterns, and the like? Do you experience a particular aura, visual or other sensory or motor problems?
- What symptoms accompany the headache? Do you suffer from nausea, vomiting, appetite disturbances, diarrhea, dizziness, sensitivity to light and sound, stuffed or running nostrils, red and tearing eye, or other symptoms?
- How do you usually behave during an attack? (The response to this question frequently offers clues to a diagnosis, as migraine patients are more likely to retreat to a dark and quiet room, while people with cluster headache usually can't sit or lie still, pacing or rocking while their headaches last.)
- What happens to you after the headache? Do you feel exhausted or exhilarated? Are you left with any other symptoms? How long do these symptoms usually last?

We find this breakdown of various types of headache extremely useful, as many patients come to us with mixed headache: a variety of intense and dull headaches that may indicate a range of diagnoses. As discussed above, taking high doses of pain relievers often causes headaches to become more frequent, so that a person who initially experienced, say, two or three intense migraines per week may eventually find herself also suffering from two or three dull headaches in the same seven-day period. Teasing out the different types of headache helps us differentiate between a patient's inborn disorder and her reactions to medication. It may also help us to identify patients whose headaches are evolving and changing.

Along with exploring the patient's own history, we like to make a *genogram,* an outline of the family history of headache, family medical history, age of siblings and parents, marital history, and offspring. Since headache usually runs in families, our having this information is important. If you are planning a trip to a new doctor or health care provider, you might prepare notes to remind yourself about whether either of your parents or any sibling or child has headaches; at what age he or she started getting them; how he or she describes the pain; and what symptoms he or she notices before, during, and after the event. Beware the headache doctor who doesn't seem interested in your family history! He or she is missing information that could be important in determining your diagnosis and treatment.

Headache Calendars

We also strongly advise patients to keep a headache calendar or diary, before and during treatment. Keeping such a calendar for a month can provide you and your doctor with valuable information about the nature of your headaches and headache triggers.

In a headache calendar, you record each headache you experience, rating it for intensity, describing accompanying symptoms, and noting how long it lasts. You also note the days you feel groggy or on the verge of a headache, and the days you enjoy having a clear head. At the same time, you record what you eat, what medication you're taking, and whether you smoked cigarettes or drank any alcohol, as well as track events at home, at work, and in your social life that might help you notice particular patterns or headache triggers. Women also note the days of their menstrual periods.

Women in particular benefit from keeping headache calendars because their female cycles are often so deeply involved in their headache patterns. A woman who keeps a headache calendar over a three-month period can track which, if any, days of the month are especially volatile for her, as well as note which headache triggers are especially dangerous on those days. For our suggested format for a headache calendar, see page 237.

If you've been keeping a headache calendar before your initial visit to a new doctor, be sure to share your calendar with her or him and see what conclusions she or he draws. (And again, beware of the doctor who is not interested in your headache calendar — she or he may not be very interested in *you*, either!)

The Physical and Neurological Examination

In addition to speaking with you about your headaches, your prospective new doctor or health care provider should give you a complete physical examination at the initial consultation. If possible, she or he should also give you a complete neurological examination and, if appropriate, refer you for certain neurological tests.

What should this physical examination include? Here are some of the elements that we observe in our intake examination:

Vital signs We take blood pressure, pulse rate, and occasionally respiration and temperature.

Head We observe the size and shape of the head, looking for signs of obvious deformity and unusual bumps.

Eyes We look to see whether we can detect any abnormalities related to the eye. We also press gently on a patient's closed lids, checking for increased pressure related to glaucoma or tenderness related to meningitis.

Jaw We feel the temperomandibular joint, checking for tenderness, and ask the patient to open and clench her jaw, to see whether doing so causes pain. Meanwhile, we check for signs of deviation of the jaw when it opens, as well as for any restriction of the jaw's range or motion. We also ask the patient whether she ever feels pain while chewing, and we listen to hear possible clicks, pops, or other evidence of malfunction.

Scalp, neck, shoulders, and spine We gently feel the head, neck, shoulders, and spine to check for tenderness and excessive muscle contraction, with particular attention to the region around the greater occipital nerves. We also watch to see whether tenderness in one area "refers" pain to other parts of the body. Since rigidity in the neck is a common symptom of meningitis, we do further tests if a patient's neck is unusually stiff.

Muscle tension Sometimes we ask a patient to extend her arm, supporting her wrist with one of our own hands. We ask her to relax her arm so that when we release it, the arm falls from its own weight. Many patients tell us that they are completely relaxed — and then when their arms are released, they don't fall. It's helpful to both us and the patient to discover the gap between their actual tension and their sense of it.

Temples We look to see whether the temporal arteries are prominent or appear swollen. We palpate the patient's temples gently to see whether they are tender or rigid.

Sinuses We palpate the sinuses to check for tenderness and swelling. Sometimes we illuminate the sinuses to determine translucence, opacity, or other factors that may help us uncover their role in headache pain.

Arteries We listen to the flow of blood through various neck arteries and feel the pulses to check for vascular problems.

Thyroid We palpate the thyroid gland to check for enlargement.

Cranial nerves A complete examination of the cranial nerves is necessary to rule out any possible organic causes of headache. (An organic cause is a problem with the body's *physical* structure, with the organism itself, as opposed to the *biochemical* problem at the root of most headaches.)

Sensory functions We make sure to test a patient's sensitivity to light touch, pinprick, cold, and vibratory sensation throughout her entire body. Migraineurs often have cold hands and feet due to constricted arteries (it's blood that warms the human body, and constricted arteries may not be carrying enough of that warming blood to the extremities).

Motor system We check many muscle groups for tone and strength, looking especially for the presence of tremors, which may be evidence of a variety of disorders, including hyperthyroidism, Parkinson's disease, multiple sclerosis, anxiety, and side effects resulting from various drugs or medications.

Cerebellar system We evaluate the function of the cerebellum — a structure in the back of the brain — and the systems it regulates by appraising the patient's gait and testing for the integrity of coordination. In addition, we check the patient's ability to move her finger between our finger and her nose and to run her heel down her shin, to walk on her toes and on her heels, and to walk heel-to-toe.

Reflexes We test all reflexes, including those of the pupils and the tendons, like the knee jerk.

Mental status A number of emotional and mental problems are frequently associated with various headache conditions, as well as with other serious organic problems, of which headaches might be only a secondary symptom. Therefore, we examine our patients for signs of depression and anxiety, including regular or frequent anxiety attacks (depression and anxiety are often associated with chronic daily headache), and obsessive or intrusive thoughts. Possible signs of post-traumatic headache include inability to concentrate; problems with memory; inability to perform simple tasks (such as subtracting a series of sevens from one hundred, or spelling five-letter words backward and forward); and inability to perform complex multiple tasks.

Overall physical examination We examine the heart and lungs, looking carefully for evidence of murmurs or irregular heartbeat (arrythmia). We also need to evaluate the patient's other medical conditions, such as asthma, hypertension, coronary artery disease, peptic ulcer, particularly with regard to prescribing headache medication. The patient may already be taking medication for other conditions that will interact in various ways with headache medication; it's also possible that headache medication may adversely affect the other conditions (e.g., migraineurs with asthma should not be given beta-blockers).

Possible overuse of drugs By the time they get to us, many patients have been overusing opiates (narcotics), barbiturates, and benzodiazepines in an effort to circumvent or abort their pain. They may also have stopped taking these medications before coming to us and be in one of the stages of withdrawal. Hence, we check for irritability, tremors, dilated pupils, and other signs of adverse reactions to drugs or withdrawal therefrom.

Ending the Initial Consultation

We believe that the end of the initial exam is even more significant than everything that came before. Here are the steps we go through at the end of each consultation, elements that you might also look for in a relationship with your new doctor:

- *We review our findings with the patient as thoroughly as possible.* Generally, we are able to make our diagnoses, or at least initial hypotheses, based on what information the first day of evaluation has yielded. We explain what we found, what our reasoning was, and if necessary, why we've recommended further tests. We then describe what treatment we recommend at this point and explain why.

- *We allow time for the patient to ask questions, voice concerns and feelings, and satisfy herself that she understands her condition and our treatment plan.* A study by Russell Packard demonstrated that patients with headache are looking not only for relief of pain but also for an explanation of the causes of their headache. Headache is a particularly difficult illness to explain, since no tests can definitely confirm its presence — they can only confirm that some other specific cause is *not* involved. Thus, we take special care in explaining to our patients our notion of headache as an inborn biochemical disorder, probably inherited, that can be triggered by a variety of factors.

- *We affirm that we consider headaches to be a valid biological disorder.* Whether or not relaxation techniques, counseling, and other psychological approaches are appropriate, headaches are ultimately the result of a *physical* problem, not a psychological one. We make sure that our patients understand our philosophy: headache is as valid a disorder as coronary artery disease, hypertension, and ulcers, even though we are not yet able to point to any biological markers to confirm its presence.

- *We review potential headache triggers: types of food, alcohol, changes in season or in the weather, schedule changes, travel, time zone changes, skipped meals, flickering lights, other sensory stimuli, and the like.* We make sure the patient understands that no one trigger inevitably sets off a headache in everyone; that each person's response to headache triggers is different; and that the response itself may change over time, either because of changes in diet and lifestyle or for no readily understandable reason. We assure the patient that we will work together to discover her particular headache triggers and enlist her help by having her keep a headache calendar (for more on headache calendars, see pages 74–75).

- *We discuss the role of stress in triggering headaches.* We point out that migraines do not result from a particular personality type, but rather from a biological predisposition to *translate* stress into headaches. However, the effects of that biological condition can sometimes be overcome or modified with aerobic exercise, relaxation techniques, or counseling designed to change one's response to stress. We then reaffirm that the problem is certainly not "all in her head" and reassure the patient that we will continue to treat her headaches, whatever is triggering them. We make sure to take the time to explore the patient's reactions to our suggestions.

- *We discuss the patient's responsibility for identifying headache triggers.* Sometimes a person can control a trigger for a headache attack, e.g., avoiding that tempting glass of red wine. Sometimes a person can identify a trigger but not control it, e.g., knowing that a sudden rise in humidity is setting off a headache. Sometimes, though, a headache may appear without any obvious triggers. Some migraines seem to occur spontaneously, following some rhythm of their own. We point out this possibility to patients, so that they don't feel they've "brought it all on themselves" or blame themselves for their painful headaches.

- *We explain our treatment plan as it relates to the other issues we've raised.* We review all drug and nondrug approaches that we think will prove helpful, taking special care to distinguish between *preventive medication*— designed to reduce or prevent headache frequency, intensity, and duration — and *abortive medication,* designed to stop a headache in progress. Many patients want medication that provides complete and immediate headache relief; if such relief isn't possible, we say so and explain why. We also let patients know that they won't necessarily be on medication for the rest of their lives and explain the procedure we plan to use for decreasing or eliminating their dosage. We explain the necessary restrictions on using abortive medication, so the patient doesn't become dependent or addicted. We make sure to leave time for patients to ask questions and express concerns.

- *We identify problems that a patient may have with overusing medication and provide her with clear guidelines for how gradually to replace problematic medications with more appropriate drug and nondrug treatments.* We also explain the phenomenon of "rebound headache," the syndrome of overusing medication to such an extent that the patient gets a headache as soon as the medication wears off.

- *Finally, we review the patient's expectations about her treatment.* Many people have the understandable wish to find a "cure" for their headaches. But unfortunately, at our present state of medical knowledge, headaches cannot be cured, they can only be controlled. True, certain headache patterns may remit or even disappear spontaneously. And a person *may* become virtually headache-free, or go from having frequent "untreatable" migraines to suffering only occasional headaches that aspirin can end. But since there is no *cure,* we can't say exactly what the outcome of treatment will be. We can only affirm that a patient *can* expect *some* relief, depending on her condition and on her willingness to participate in her own treatment.

Initiating a Partnership

Remember, if your new physician or other provider doesn't volunteer the information you want, feel free to ask. If he or she doesn't open a topic for discussion that you're concerned about, *you* give it a try. Volunteer your concerns or state your expectations and see what kind of response you get. Give your healer a chance to enter into a true partnership with you.

However, if he or she doesn't take that chance, despite your best efforts to be open and responsible, you might want to consider looking further. If you're ready to take an active role in treating your headaches, you deserve a partner who supports your commitment and enthusiasm.

CONTINUING YOUR NEW PARTNERSHIP

The Need for Follow-up Visits

If you do decide to start seeing a new doctor or health care provider, what can you expect after that first consultation? We believe that the subsequent ongoing follow-up visits are key, since most headaches are also chronic and ongoing. It's highly unlikely that the first visit will yield the perfect combination of drug and nondrug therapies that will swiftly resolve the problem. Time to experiment with different possibilities, to try out long-term nondrug treatments (such as changes in diet or increased aerobic exercise), and to observe the long-term effects of medication is an integral part of a successful treatment. Both doctor and patient should be prepared for several return visits, averaging three to four per year.

The frequency of these visits depends on the progress of the patient and on the strength of any drugs that may have been prescribed. We generally schedule our first follow-up visit within two to four weeks of the initial consultation.

What Happens at a Follow-up Visit?

The purpose of the follow-up visit is to review progress, based on the patient's verbal reports and on a closer look at her headache calendar. We can't stress too strongly the importance of the calendar. Pain is obviously a subjective experience, and what a person remembers and feels most intensely at the time of the doctor's visit is not necessarily the whole picture.

For example, we once treated a patient who suffered from chronic daily headache. At her initial visit she reported that she experienced mild to moderate waxing and waning pain every single day, along with periodic episodes of more intense migraines that virtually incapacitated her for twenty-four hours at a time. We prescribed beta-blockers and asked her to come back for a follow-up visit. At that time, she told us that the medication had obviously failed, since her daily headache pain was unchanged. If that had been all the data we had, we would probably have upped the dosage of her medication or perhaps switched to a stronger drug. When we reviewed her headache calendar with her, however, it came out that, although her mild to moderate daily pain remained unchanged, she had had no more incapacitating migraines. In fact, then, the beta-blocker *had* been successful in combating her migraine attacks, even though it was apparently not effective in reducing her daily pain. This information was of prime importance in determining her future treatment.

Besides reviewing the overall effectiveness (or lack thereof) of treatment, a follow-up visit is also the occasion for discussing whether the patient is suffering from any side effects, for taking the patient's vital signs and reexamining her as necessary, and for exploring the patient's general sense of well-being. We also review possible nondrug approaches to the patient's headache, including diet, exercise, stress management, lifestyle changes, and the like. Finally, we find out about upcoming important events in the patient's life, such as a family visit, a major work deadline, or even a holiday. This information then gives us the basis for later exploring with the patient how she handled whatever headache triggers might have been part of the event.

Phone Calls between Visits

We find between-visit phone calls an extremely important part of headache treatment. The most obvious use of a phone call, of course, is to report an emergency. However, it may also be important for patients to alert us to disturbing side effects that do not constitute an emergency but that may necessitate either phone consultation or a moved-up office visit. Naturally, major changes in preventive medication should not be made over the phone, but a patient who is concerned about side effects should not have to wait two to four weeks to express her concerns.

Maintaining the Doctor-Patient Relationship

Over the weeks and months that follow the initial visit, both the doctor and the patient have certain responsibilities. As we see it, the doctor's responsibilities include the following:

- monitoring the patient's response to treatment
- exploring new treatment options, if necessary
- suggesting nondrug treatments

- being responsive to the patient's concerns about side effects, lifestyle, and other issues
- being aware of changes in headache, even in long-term patients (after all, a person with chronic daily headache might *also* develop an organic problem that causes headaches)

The patient, on the other hand, is responsible for the following:

- keeping appointments
- following an agreed-upon treatment plan
- taking only medication prescribed by us or that we have been fully informed of
- holding onto prescriptions
- keeping phone calls to the necessary minimum, rather than using them as an occasion for counseling or as a substitute for missed visits

In our opinion, the treatment that has the best chance of success is that which is based on doctor and patient each behaving responsibly. If either party is frustrated with the behavior of the other, it's important to share those feelings and clear the air. If either party is unwilling to do this — if a doctor refuses to take reports of side effects seriously, say, or if a patient insists on getting pain medication from more than one doctor — then the relationship will probably not produce an effective treatment.

EMERGENCY ROOM VISITS

Sometimes, especially in the early stages of a new treatment, it becomes necessary for patients to visit the emergency room to respond to an overwhelmingly painful headache.

Our patients have told us of rude or dismissive treatment on such visits. Perhaps the medical staff at the hospital they visit aren't familiar with the latest research on headache. Perhaps the staff doesn't consider headache a truly valid biological ailment or one that merits their serious attention in the midst of more pressing emergencies. Perhaps, too, they have had bad experiences with patients feigning illness as a semilegal way of obtaining narcotics. The residue of these experiences and attitudes can result in a very bad experience for the headache sufferer, who is already upset enough at being driven by pain to seek emergency care.

In our opinion, the best way to circumvent this problem is to provide our patients with a written treatment plan specifying what care we would suggest in the event of an emergency. For example, we give our patients cards suggesting that emergency room care for a severe migraine attack should include three separate injections:

- D.H.E. 45   1 mg   IM
- Phenergan   50 mg   IM
- Decadron   4 mg   IM

We date and sign the cards and suggest that patients keep them in their wallets for emergency use. We suggest that you, too, ask your doctor for a written treatment plan that includes suggested measures for emergency care.

THE DOCTOR-PATIENT RELATIONSHIP: RESPONSIBILITIES AND REWARDS

The model of medical care that we outline in this chapter demands a great deal more work on both sides than the traditional paternalistic model. Doctors must spend time and energy focusing on each patient's individual needs, feelings, and responses; patients must seek doctors with whom they can communicate, must keep accurate track of their own behavior, and must participate actively in all aspects of their treatment.

We believe that although the responsibilities of such a relationship are great, the rewards are even greater. In our experience, a woman who knows what to expect from treatment, from her doctor, and from herself is able to find the doctor or other health care provider who is right for her. She is able to work with that healer to prevent and manage her headache pain. Perhaps most importantly, she learns more about her body, her emotions, and her life choices; becomes aware of how to better care for herself; and, ultimately, experiences a sense of empowerment and control over her life.

CHAPTER 4

Migraine and Menstruation

WOMEN, MENSTRUATION, AND MIGRAINE: TAKING THE COMPLAINT SERIOUSLY

IN CHILDHOOD, boys are slightly more likely to get migraines than girls. As soon as children hit puberty, however, the ratio shifts strongly in favor of women, three to one. Approximately 33 percent of female migraineurs start getting headaches at or soon after menarche (the onset of menstruation at puberty). And some 60 percent of women who get migraines report getting them during the days just before, during, or just after their periods. Twenty-five percent of these women say they never get migraines at any other time. Some women also get migraines exclusively during ovulation.

Clearly, there is a correlation between the female hormonal cycle and migraine headache. As already discussed, migraines are basically the result of a biochemical disorder in the brain that responds to various migraine triggers. Apparently, one of those triggers has to do with the fluctuating levels of female hormones that take place during menstruation.

Of course, the hormonal cycle can't be the *only* significant migraine trigger, since prepubescent girls and males of all ages get migraines too. Apparently, though, the complicated biological process of menstruation can set off the almost as complicated biochemical process that produces a headache.

For years women who suffered from menstrual migraine had to endure a kind of double whammy. Not only did many doctors and scientists not take migraine seriously as a valid biological disorder, they also tended to be relatively uninterested in women's experience of their menstrual cycles.

Today we know better. Although much about both migraine and menstruation remains to be understood, we are developing a far more sophisticated understanding of the range and nature of interactions between these two processes. This understanding is important, because the more we know, the more we realize how much we *don't* know. Some studies suggest that the menstrual cycle itself can be a migraine trigger for many women. Other studies, however, distinguish between women who get headaches *only* during certain times of the month and women who *also* get headaches during those times; apparently, different types of treatment are successful with each group. Still other studies question the notion of a unique menstrual migraine; researchers who have conducted these studies maintain that all migraines are essentially the same, no matter what triggered them.

In this chapter, we explore the latest scientific research on the relationship between migraine and menstruation. But because this area has been so little studied in the past, a great deal still remains to be done. Possibly by the time this book has gone to press, new discoveries will have been made and new treatments will be available. At least, though, doctors and scientists are now taking seriously the importance of understanding a woman's menstrual cycle in diagnosing and treating her migraines.

THE MENSTRUAL CYCLE

To understand the relationship between migraine and menstruation, you need to understand the menstrual cycle itself. Although identifying "the" cycle is a bit arbitrary, since the process is continuous, scientists generally speak of the menstrual cycle as beginning on the first day of menstruation, Day 1, and ending on the day before the next menses begins, Day −1.

The menstrual cycle represents a series of biological events that enable women to bear children. Each event is triggered by a specific combination of *hormones,* substances secreted by the body's various *glands,* which travel in the blood stream to affect other glands. The hormones triggered by each event in turn inspire the release of other hormones. Or, in some cases, the release of one hormone inhibits the production or release of another. This complicated system of interlocking biological events combines to produce the following process:

- a follicle within the ovary grows
- the follicle releases its egg — *ovulation*
- the follicle becomes a *corpus luteum,* a mass of yellow tissue formed by the ruptured follicle whose egg has been released
- the endometrial lining of the uterus grows thicker, preparing to nourish a fertilized egg
- if no egg is fertilized, the endometrial lining becomes the bloody menstrual discharge
- another follicle begins to grow, ready to begin the next cycle

THE PREMENSTRUAL PHASE

For the menstrual cycle to begin, several parts of the body must coordinate their activities, each releasing the appropriate level of hormones at the appropriate time:

- The *hypothalamus* secretes the gonadotropin-releasing hormone (GnRH). It in turn works on the pituitary gland.

- The *pituitary* gland secretes the glycoproteins luteinizing hormone (LH) and follicle-stimulating hormone (FSH).
- The *ovary* secretes estrogens (female sex hormones) and progesterone (a substance from which either female or male sex hormones may be synthesized).

The entire process of hormone secretion is regulated by a number of chemicals in the brain, including *serotonin,* which, as already discussed, is involved with the biochemical process that produces migraine, as well as with depression, anxiety, sleep disturbances, and our general sense of — or lack of — well-being. *Noradrenaline* is also a key chemical in this process. (For more on noradrenaline's role in diet, insulin production, and migraine, see Chapter 7.) Other neurotransmitters are also involved, including *opioids* and a chemical known as *CRH.*

The process begins, then, when these various neurotransmitters "instruct" the hypothalamus to secrete GnRH, which stimulates the pituitary to secrete LH and FSH, in turn stimulating the ovaries to secrete estrogen and progesterone. Estrogen and progesterone go on to regulate the pituitary, moderating the amounts of LH and FSH that are secreted; they also regulate the hypothalamus's production of GnRH.

Meanwhile, the neurotransmitters we've identified are playing contradictory roles. Norepinephrine is stimulating the hypothalamus to produce *more* GnRH, while the opioids and CRH are "instructing" the hypothalamus to produce *less.*

As you can see, even this initial stage of the menstrual process is extremely complicated, with a variety of hormones balancing each other out in their instructions to various other parts of the body. Throughout the menstrual process, the levels of estrogen and other hormones rise and fall, with various effects and countereffects at each stage. The menstrual cycle is a carefully coordinated sequence of changes that may be interrupted by subtle "miscues," such as extreme weight loss, excessive exercise, or even unusual amounts of emotional stress, which in some cases can signal the body to stop menstruation. This interruption occurs because malnutrition, the excessive depletion of body fat, or unusually high levels of exercise all produce extra *endorphins,* the body's natural narcotic. Endorphins, which desensitize us to pain and produce a natural sense of well-being, also seem to inhibit the menstrual cycle, producing *amenorrhea,* or the absence of menses.

In men, by contrast, hormone levels remain relatively constant, so that while men are certainly affected by weight loss, exercise, and stress, their hormonal processes apparently are not. This difference may be one of the reasons why women are so much more susceptible to migraine than men are: the *changes* in hormonal levels that constitute the menstrual cycle cause major changes in blood vessels, blood pressure, and in the body's tendency to retain fluids, as well as changes in a number of other areas, like the brain itself.

Some hormones even play two different roles within the process. Various levels of progesterone, for example, initially facilitate sexual behavior and later inhibit it, explaining why women often experience various surges and drops in sexual excitability throughout the monthly cycle.

Progesterone also affects the body's experience of anxiety and depression, at least among women who suffer from *late luteal phase dysphoric disorder* (LLPDD), a collection of symptoms commonly known as the *premenstrual syndrome* (PMS) that comes from the hormonal changes preceding menstruation. LLPDD is named after the time of the month when the disorder takes place — while the follicle is discharging its corpus luteum in the ovary, a time known as the late luteal phase. Women with LLPDD have reported that their anxiety or depression increases progressively during the late luteal phase, resolves rapidly when menstruation begins, and then remains stable until their progesterone rises again during their next late luteal phase. Other symptoms of LLPDD include backache, breast swelling and tenderness, lethargy, crying spells, difficulty in thinking, nausea — and sometimes premenstrual migraine.

Perhaps surprisingly, the hormonal chain of events that leads up to menstruation and the symptoms of premenstrual syndrome seem to be two relatively separate processes. We know this because women whose periods have been delayed by various medical treatments nevertheless get PMS at the time of the month when they would normally have gotten it, even though the timing of their actual menstruation has been artificially changed. We now suspect that PMS symptoms, including premenstrual migraine, represent an autonomous disorder, linked to but independent of the menstrual cycle. However, artificial suppression of ovulation does seem to result in the remission of PMS symptoms.

Clearly, the variety of hormonal events going on throughout the menstrual cycle makes it extremely difficult to disentangle various aspects of the process from one another. We do know, however, that premenstrual migraine and menstrual migraine are two distinct syndromes, responding to different hormonal events — and susceptible to different types of treatment.

MENSTRUAL MIGRAINE

If the symptoms associated with premenstrual migraine are those of PMS, the main symptom associated with menstrual migraine is *dysmenorrhea,* or a painful period. Some women get migraines only during their menses, while others may experience menses as a migraine trigger, along with other triggers that set off headaches throughout the month.

What is it about menstruation that acts as a migraine trigger? Researchers are not yet able to answer that question, but we suspect that the main culprit is the *withdrawal of estrogen.* Low levels of estrogen in themselves don't seem to trigger migraines (nor do high levels); rather, the process of *falling* estrogen seems to set off the migraine. In any case, the greatest fluctuations of estrogen levels take place just before and during menses; these are also the two times of the cycle most associated with migraine. These levels also fluctuate, to a lesser extent, at midcycle; and migraine may occur at ovulation as well.

The fluctuations in estrogen levels produce many biochemical changes that might account for menstrual migraine. We'll take a look at just one type of substance that may be involved: prostaglandins.

Prostaglandins and the Uterus

Prostaglandins sensitize the body's response to pain and stimulate the nervous system to produce inflammation. Various prostaglandins seem to be related to various types of pain. One type, prostacyclin, when injected into experimental subjects, produced a dull, throbbing headache. Another type, PGE_1, produced migraine-like headaches and abdominal cramps. Yet another type, PGF_2, produced cramping, diarrhea, nausea, flushing, fainting, and the inability to concentrate.

During the menstrual cycle, estrogen and progesterone stimulate the endometrium to release prostaglandins, particularly PGE_1 (apparently related to migraine and cramping) and PGF_2 (apparently related to the symptoms of premenstrual migraine and PMS). Researchers note that patients who suffer from menstrual difficulties such as cramping have shown increased concentrations of prostaglandins in their menstrual discharges. These same prostaglandins may also have been the trigger for menstrual migraine.

DOES MENSTRUAL MIGRAINE REALLY EXIST?

Many researchers have come to accept the notion of a distinct type of migraine known as "menstrual migraine."

They point out that some 16 percent of women with migraine get headaches only during their periods, and these women, too, are likely to have started getting their headaches at the time of their menarche. These are also the women whose headaches ease during pregnancy, suggesting that their only headache trigger is the menstrual cycle.

On the other hand, some researchers point out that there are no specific clinical characteristics that can distinguish migraine triggered by hormones from migraine triggered by other sources. Like all migraine, menstrual migraine is characterized by a throbbing pain on one side of the head, nausea and vomiting, sensitivity to light and sound, and a duration from four to twenty-four hours. Some menstrual migraines are heralded by an aura, just like regular classical migraines; others are not, just like regular common migraines. These researchers are skeptical of the notion of a separate category of menstrual migraine. (For more on migraine types and symptoms, see Chapter 2.)

We ourselves believe that there is value in identifying this category because women who get headaches only in relation to their hormonal cycles appear to be far more difficult to treat. Whereas thermal biofeedback has proved enormously helpful to many migraineurs, it is significantly less helpful for women with exclusively menstrual migraine. (For more about biofeedback, see Chapter 8.)

A study of 720 women with migraine, conducted in Italy by researcher Giovanni Nattero, found that women who got headaches exclusively during their periods differed considerably from women who got headaches throughout the month. The two groups of women seemed to have completely different patterns with regard to family background, headache histories, experience of premenstrual stress, and headache-related reactions to menstruation and pregnancy.

Indeed, some scientists have proposed that menstrual migraine is more appropriately diagnosed as part of a complex syndrome of menstrually related difficulties (of which one is PMS/LLMDD) affecting the body's metabolism, nervous system, circulatory system, and neurologically generated emotions (e.g., anxiety, depression, confusion, inability to concentrate). In these scientists' view, menstrual migraine is a subset of menstrual problems, rather than a subset of migraine per se.

Clearly, much research on menstrual migraine remains to be done. Meanwhile, however, women and their doctors would benefit from an awareness of the special features of menstrual migraine.

MIGRAINE, HORMONES, AND YOUR LIVER

The organ of the body charged with breaking down excess estrogen or progesterone is the liver. The liver generally functions as the body's purifier; it must detoxify any alcohol, nicotine, caffeine, or preservatives that a person ingests, as well as break down fats. A toxic liver, such as one overworked by too much alcohol, may not be able to break down estrogen or progesterone effectively. Such ineffective breakdown may translate into hormone imbalances and, once again, into migraine, as well as PMS and other menstrual difficulties. (For more on the role of your liver and your diet in migraine, see Chapter 7.)

RESPONDING TO MENSTRUALLY RELATED MIGRAINE

Exercise

One of the best ways to respond to menstrually related migraine is to get plenty of aerobic exercise, especially during the time between ovulation and your period. Aerobic exercise produces endorphins and releases stress — effects that can help combat the factors contributing to menstrual and premenstrual migraine.

Diet

Many foods are implicated in triggering migraine. Sometimes these foods are precisely what women crave during their menstrual or premenstrual times: chocolate, cold cuts, nuts, aged cheese, and salty foods. Generally, foods containing tyramine (red wine, aged cheese, liver, figs, and avocado), phenylethylamine (chocolate), and nitrites (bologna, salami, and hot dogs) — while always dangerous for migraineurs — are particularly dangerous for migraineurs who suffer from menstrual or premenstrual migraine. (For a more complete list of migraine-triggering foods, see page 138 in Chapter 7.)

If you have menstrually related headaches, you might cut these foods out of your diet during the week or two before your period and see how you respond. If this temporary abstinence helps and you miss the foods, you might try bringing them back one at a time to see which ones are the headache triggers.

Too much caffeine or withdrawal from it may be a migraine trigger at any time of the month. As a vasoconstrictor, it narrows your blood vessels, so that they can push the blood through faster. Caffeine has the ability to wake you up. Like exercise, it gets your blood moving, both raising your body temperature and making you feel more alert. But when the caffeine wears off, your blood vessels dilate again. If you're a migraineur, this dilation could bring on a headache.

As with the other foods described here, coffee or caffeinated teas and colas in moderation may be fine for you during the rest of the month. But during sensitive times, it might bring on a headache. If you're not ready to give up caffeine entirely, see if you can limit your intake to one cup of coffee or two cups of tea per day, at least during the week or so before your period and during your period itself. Some people find that taking vitamin B supplements helps combat the symptoms of caffeine withdrawal.

Of course, if you're used to drinking a lot of caffeine, the week before your period is *not* the time to start giving it up! Caffeine withdrawal can also bring on headaches, so save it for the week after your period, when your system has more reserves to deal with the strain.

There is some evidence that migraine may be linked to hypoglycemia, or low blood sugar. According to some researchers, headaches are more frequently triggered in hypoglycemics, because they produce excessive amounts of insulin. The abnormally high levels of insulin constantly threaten to lower a hypoglycemic's blood sugar below an acceptable level, bringing on a migraine. Since processed sugar and highly sweet foods are most likely to trigger an insulin rush, especially on an empty stomach, they also pose the greatest danger to a person's blood sugar levels.

Therefore, if you suffer from menstrually related migraine, you might try to cut out sweets for the week or two before your period. Be especially careful not to eat something sweet, like a Danish or a sweet roll, first thing in the morning; and don't let a piece of cake or a muffin be a midmorning or midafternoon snack. If you must eat sweets, save them for dessert, after you've already had a nutritious meal that will help keep your blood sugar at an acceptable level. It's best, though, if you can try cutting out sweets at this time and see what effect it has.

You might also want to find out if you really *do* suffer from hypoglycemia. There's a chance that you have this problem if you feel irritable or panicky about missing a meal or if you feel anxious or upset within an hour or so after eating something sweet. If these are indeed your reactions, you may not have noticed them until now, or you may never have associated these reactions with your diet. You might try eating small meals of protein and carbohydrates regularly and frequently. Some people with this problem must eat every two hours! Some people also supply themselves with a light snack before bed — some crackers and possibly some mild cheese — to guard against blood sugar levels falling during the night and bringing on a headache in the morning.

In any case, the week before your period is the worst possible time to miss meals, to start a crash diet, or to cut back on carbohydrates (whole grains, pasta, potatoes). Some studies have suggested that the hormonal fluctuations of the menstrual cycle also bring fluctuations in blood sugar, so eating regularly is important. And the carbohydrates help you cope with the anxiety and depression that may be biochemically induced at this time.

Generally, both migraineurs and women with menstrually related problems benefit from a diet low in sugar, salt, fat, caffeine, and preservatives and from a diet high in proteins and complex carbohydrates (pasta and bread). You may not realize how good such a diet makes you feel until you've tried it!

Alcohol is another possible migraine trigger, particularly around the time of your period. In addition to its biochemical effect on the body, which can directly trigger a headache, alcohol is a toxin, which the liver must then purify. Liquor that you can handle at other times of the month may be too much for you just before or during menses.

Once again, we suggest cutting liquor out of your premenstrual and early menstrual diet. If doing so helps, you've learned something more about how to care for yourself. (For more on migraine and diet, see Chapter 7.)

Vitamins

We often suggest that women take vitamin B_6 in doses of 50 to 100 mg per day just before, during, and just after menstruation. This vitamin is a natural diuretic, so it will help stabilize your fluid levels despite the effects of estrogen. Stress, caffeine, and birth control pills all deplete the body's supply of B_6, so it's important to replace it as you can. It also helps in a biochemical reaction that increases the amount of serotonin in the brain.

Women who suffer from PMS may also find it helpful to take vitamin E supplements of 400 IU per day (considerably higher than the recommended dose of 10 mg). We further suggest that our patients with menstrual migraine take a multivitamin and 200 to 400 mg of vitamin B_2 every day.

On the other hand, we don't suggest that you exceed the recommended daily allowance of vitamins without the supervision of a qualified health care provider. The megadoses of vitamin B have been known to have toxic results in some women with migraine.

Recent studies have revealed that many migraineurs may suffer from a deficiency of magnesium in the cerebral cortex (a part of the brain). We suggest 400 mg of magnesium to reduce both the severity of PMS symptoms and the duration and intensity of premenstrual migraine.

Self-Awareness

The great thing about understanding your body is that you can learn how to give yourself what you need. Paying attention to yourself allows you to recognize the signs that a headache may be coming on, to be aware of what foods and beverages may put a strain on your system, or to sense when you need a vigorous walk or an hour of aerobics to help release the day's accumulated stress. As you think further about your headaches and your monthly cycle, you may realize some other headache triggers that bother you only during your critical time of the month.

You may find that eliminating one headache trigger helps you tolerate others, e.g., staying out of smoke-filled rooms while you're premenstrual means you can get away with an occasional glass of white wine, or exercising vigorously for the two weeks before your period means you can have that brownie you've been craving. On the other hand, you may discover that giving up caffeine, sweets, and alcohol brings you not only relief from headaches but a new sense of well-being all month long. We and your doctors can only share with you our understanding of potential headache triggers. Figuring out which ones affect you and to what extent you must avoid them is up to you.

MEDICATING MENSTRUALLY RELATED MIGRAINE

Both premenstrual and menstrual migraines are difficult to treat, but they can be treated. However, each condition tends to respond to different medication, so it's important to distinguish between the two. Make sure you and your doctor are working together with detailed, specific information about your headaches' timing, your symptoms, and other details about your menstrual cycle, so that he or she can make a proper diagnosis.

Some nonsteroidal anti-inflammatory drugs (such as naproxen sodium and ketoprofen may bring relief to women suffering from menstrually related migraine. Other helpful medications include Bellergal, Midrin, Cafergot, D.H.E. 45, and Imitrex.

Women who get headaches only during their menses may be treated with antidepressants, beta-blockers, calcium channel blockers, or methysergide. Women who are taking these medications for headache throughout the month may be prescribed increased doses of them for the week or two before their periods.

Generally, we recommend preventive medication when a woman is getting three or more attacks per month, if these headache attacks are prolonged, and particularly if the headaches are not responding to abortive medication. However, as with all medication plans, women and their doctors must make sure that the woman is not overusing pain relievers, as that can in itself cause headaches.

Sometimes women find that their medication is in fact successful in eliminating all of their headaches — except those associated with their menses. In some cases, a reasonable goal for eliminating menstrually related migraine might be a 50 percent reduction in headaches with no intolerable side effects.

As a rule, medication should begin at the lowest dose possible, both to guard against side effects and to see if the body is in fact responsive to the lower level of medication. However, medication may have to be increased based on the woman's response.

In some cases, it's possible to reduce medication in three to six months and eventually even to eliminate it. Once again, if complete elimination of medication is important to you, be sure to share this treatment goal with your doctor.

HORMONAL THERAPIES

By and large, we consider hormonal therapies a last resort. After all, the hormonal fluctuations of the menstrual cycle are complicated enough on their own! However, if all other medications fail and a woman is still suffering from incapacitating headaches during her menses, we then consider hormonal therapy.

Successful hormonal therapy for menstrual migraine has included the use of estrogens, estrogen antagonists (substances that would reduce the level of estrogens), estrogens in combination with testosterone (a male sex hormone), and prolactin-release inhibitors. (*Prolactin* is a substance released by the pituitary gland during the menstrual cycle that many researchers believe is implicated as a migraine trigger.) Progesterone by itself does not seem effective in treating menstrual migraine and often worsens headache.

The theory behind using estrogen therapy is that migraines are triggered by falling levels of estrogen during the late luteal phase (the premenstrual time when the empty follicle releases its corpus luteum in the ovary). Thus, "replacing" the lost estrogen can keep hormone levels high, preventing the onset of a migraine.

Various versions of estrogen replacement have been tried starting four days before the period till the end of menses, with varying levels of success. An estrogen patch allows for relatively stable levels of estrogen. Some doctors have also administered a cutaneous gel (*cutaneous* means "on the skin"), as well as tablets of estradiol (Estrace), a form of estrogen; these seem to keep estrogen levels relatively stable.

Danazol (Danocrine), which suppresses the pituitary and the ovary, and tamoxifen (Nolvadex), which blocks estrogen, may be effective in treating menstrual migraine. Tamoxifen is particularly good for menstrual migraines that have resisted other types of treatment, but it does induce a medical menopause if given regularly, and causes hot flashes.

SURGERY

One treatment that is *not* effective as a response to menstrual migraine is hysterectomy, the surgical removal of the uterus. However, to our surprise, some doctors are again advocating this procedure for their menstrual migraineurs. Other doctors are suggesting ovariectomy, the removal of the ovaries.

Although there may be some anecdotal evidence that these procedures have had some beneficial effect on migraine, they are followed by high-dose estrogen supplements after the operation. Thus, there is no way of telling whether the improvement in the headaches was caused by the operation or by the far less radical procedure of administering continuous estrogen. In our opinion, it is entirely possible that the use of estrogen after the operation was enough to account for the positive results.

Furthermore, none of the studies cited to support this procedure could be placebo-controlled (that is, there is no way to compare women who actually had the operation with women who only *thought* they had it). But women with PMS are known to be extremely sensitive to placebo: In one experiment, for example, women who were given estradiol patches and women who were given placebo patches showed the same positive responses for three entire months. It was not until six months had passed that the women with the real patches showed results that differed from the women with placebos. Thus, it seems quite possible that the women who seemed to respond to hysterectomies and ovariectomies were only responding to the *idea* of such a radical (and therefore supposedly effective) procedure.

To us, the very idea that an operation with such far-reaching physical and psychological consequences could even be considered as a treatment, particularly in the absence of any long-term, follow-up, or controlled studies to suggest its effectiveness, is absurd. It is an unfortunate example of the tendency of some doctors to treat women as a collection of symptoms rather than as whole human beings.

MENSTRUAL MIGRAINE: A LAST WORD

It's always difficult to speak about the psychological or emotional factors in migraine without making it sound as if "it's all in your head." At the risk of repeating ourselves: Migraine springs from a valid biochemical disorder, and menstrual migraine — along with its emotional components of anxiety and depression — likewise has biological roots in the nervous, hormonal, and circulatory systems.

However, that being said, it's certainly true that women's feelings about themselves, their bodies, and their lives are involved in their responses to migraine in general and to menstrual migraine in particular. Do you feel that it's your right to take a few hours off to cope with menstrual cramps, or do you believe you must keep going at top speed under all circumstances? Are you willing to give yourself special, soothing treats to combat premenstrual fatigue and depression, or do you feel angry with yourself for being "weak" or "needy"? Do the people around you support your female presence in their lives, or do coworkers, friends, or family members have difficulty dealing with your womanly body and spirit? And, perhaps most important of all, are you genuinely interested in entering into a partnership with your body, in which you listen to what you feel and what you need and respond to the best of your ability, or does your body, and particularly your female cycle, seem like an enemy, an unknown territory, a treacherous land mine — anything but a beloved aspect of yourself?

Difficulties with your body, your feelings, and your treatment by others haven't created your headaches. But they may be triggering them or, at the very least, keeping you from taking action that may prevent them or reduce their pain. We strongly urge you, as part of any treatment, to allow yourself some time to think about these issues, to listen to what your body may be telling you about yourself and your life. Keep a private journal, take time out for some long walks in a peaceful place, draw pictures of your feelings, or talk things over with a trusted friend. If painful or exciting discoveries come up that you'd like to explore further, consider finding a therapist to help you work things out.

Women in our society face a variety of assaults and demands, and are often given all too little support to deal with them. Frequently, women are expected to internalize their own exploitation, cheerfully accepting lower pay, willingly doing more than their share of the household duties. If pressures like these are related to your menstrual or premenstrual migraines, listen to what your body is telling you — and find a way to get what you need.

CHAPTER 5

Migraine, Pregnancy, and Oral Contraceptives

ALTHOUGH HORMONES PLAY A KEY ROLE in triggering migraine for many women, the hormonal activity of pregnancy helps bring headache relief to many women.

On the other hand, some women experience the first bad headaches of their lives during pregnancy, and others get their first, or worst, migraines soon after giving birth for the first time. With pregnancy, as with menstruation, there are no straightforward answers or simple explanations, only a set of basic principles that each woman and her health care provider can use to illuminate that woman's individual situation.

Likewise, the experience of taking oral contraceptives, whether in the form of birth control pills or morning-after pills, varies from woman to woman, depending on the particular pill involved, the woman's hormonal activity, and probably such other factors as the woman's diet, exercise patterns, life circumstances, and emotional responses.

A longtime complaint of the women's health movement has been that too little medical and research attention has been paid to the basic biological events of women's lives: menstruation, pregnancy, and menopause. This scant attention has extended to the more specialized field of how migraine relates to these experiences. Nonetheless, although we still know all too little, we do know something. In this chapter, we describe the basic biology of how migraine interacts with pregnancy and oral contraception, as well as discuss the latest discoveries in drug and nondrug treatment for migraine during pregnancy.

ORAL CONTRACEPTIVES AND MIGRAINE

Both the birth control pill and the morning-after pill are composed of hormones designed to intervene in the normal hormonal interactions that make up a woman's menstrual cycle. As noted in Chapter 4, this cycle is enormously complicated, with continually shifting levels of hormones that react differently at different points in the cycle. Women with migraine seem to be particularly sensitive to these fluctuations, which can frequently trigger a headache or put such a strain on the system that the woman becomes more sensitive than usual to other headache triggers, such as alcohol or foods containing tyramine.

Thus, hormone treatments of any kind can pose particular difficulties for women with migraine. Birth control pills are like other hormone treatments in this regard and, for that reason, are not generally recommended for female migraineurs.

Birth Control Pills

The oral contraceptives most commonly used in the United States mainly consist of some combination of synthetic forms of estrogen and progesterone, usually taken for twenty-one days each month. The contraceptives' main function is to prevent ovulation. As discussed in Chapter 4, the normal monthly cycle includes surges of hormones from both the hypothalamus and the pituitary, stimulating the growth of a follicle in the ovary and the release of its egg. The synthetic estrogen and progesterone in a sense "fool" the hypothalamus and the pituitary into thinking that it's a different point in the cycle, so that they don't release the hormones necessary for fertility (FSH and LH). Another type of oral contraceptive involves only the use of a synthetic progesterone, which inhibits only the pituitary from releasing its hormones. Most women respond to birth control pills with an increased tendency to migraine and other headache. Some 50 percent of the women who start on oral contraception without ever having had a migraine may become migraine-prone after taking the pill, particularly if there has been a family history of migraine.

We don't know exactly why women have this reaction, given that migraine is caused by an inborn biochemical disorder that presumably is present in a migraineur whether she takes the pill or not. However, perhaps a pre-existing tendency to this disorder (as suggested by the family history of migraine) is exacerbated by the oral contraceptive's interference with the woman's normal hormonal fluctuations.

People who are already getting headaches may experience more intense, more frequent, or longer-lasting pain, sometimes associated with neurological symptoms. Some women show a particular tendency to get headaches on the days when they are not taking the pill, i.e., the days just prior to and during their periods. This is a particularly vulnerable time for female migraineurs anyway, because of the hormonal fluctuations (a drop in estrogen levels).

On the other hand, some women's headaches are not affected when they take oral contraceptives. And a few actually experience relief from headache when they go on the pill. It's also true that the newer oral contraceptives available now have considerably lower doses of estrogen than those that first came on the market twenty years ago. The lower-dose pills seem to cause less headache pain.

In any case, if a woman is going to develop migraines in response to the pill, she'll probably do so within the first several months. Some women go on to suffer more severe migraines years later, possibly because other triggering factors have entered their lives or less likely because of the accumulated hormonal interference of the contraception.

Women who get migraines from the pill usually stop getting them when they stop taking the pill but the improvement may not be significant for up to six months.

For many years, studies suggested that women with migraine who took oral contraceptives were putting themselves at significant risk for stroke. We have long known that both migraine and oral contraception were associated with stroke, so the two in combination seemed particularly dangerous. If a woman smoked as well as having migraine and being on the pill, she seemed to be in even greater danger: of stroke, heart attack, and cancer.

A few years ago the Collaborative Group for the Study of Stroke in Young Women issued what they considered to be a definitive report, stating that "our data do not confirm previous reports suggesting that migraine may increase the risk of stroke in women using [oral contraceptives]." In our opinion, however, the relationship between migraine, oral contraceptives, and stroke remains controversial. We almost never prescribe birth control pills for women with migraine; indeed, if they are on the pill, we often urge them to find another form of contraception, especially if their headaches are worsening.

The biggest factor in increasing stroke in female migraineurs is smoking — ten times the risk. Quit! Please!

The Morning-After Pill

Although morning-after pills are taken very infrequently— they must be taken soon after unprotected intercourse, to discourage an unwanted pregnancy — they too pose the risk of cancer, heart attack, and stroke. Certainly no one should rely on this pill (diethylstilbestrol, or DES) as a major form of birth control, but migraineurs should be especially wary.

Taking DES once or twice after an unplanned sexual encounter might do nothing worse than trigger another migraine, but taking it more regularly poses a truly unacceptable risk.

A WORD ABOUT NORPLANT

Norplant is a series of tubular implants beneath the skin of the upper arm designed to continually release a form of progesterone in order to inhibit pregnancy. However, the side effects of this device include irregular menstrual bleeding and headache, which occur in approximately 5 to 20 percent of the women who use Norplant. In fact, the two most common reasons women gave for removing the device were headache and menstrual disturbance.

PREGNANCY

One of the most upsetting aspects of pregnancy for the migraineur is the prospect of not being able to take any migraine medication for nine months! This inability is particularly problematic for the many female migraineurs who experience some increased headache pain during the first trimester. Fortunately, many women find new relief from migraine during pregnancy, particularly during the second and third trimesters. In some cases, women have reported being completely without headaches while pregnant (or while in the later stages of pregnancy), for the first time they can remember.

Apparently women's reactions to pregnancy may vary, depending upon her previous headache patterns. In one 1990 study, researchers found that some 7 percent of women who had gotten headaches exclusively during their menstrual periods reported that pregnancy made their headaches worse. Up to 15 percent of the women who got headaches through-

out the month found that pregnancy worsened their headaches. For women like these, there are some medications that
may be given during pregnancy if absolutely necessary, such
as acetaminophen (Tylenol), alone or with codeine and
injectable meperidine (Demerol), often given with an antinausea medicine.

The Biology of Pregnancy

What is it about pregnancy that affects headaches one way
or the other? As with the relationship between migraine and
menstruation, there's much about this topic that we still don't
know. Certainly, estrogen, the female sex hormone, is involved in some way. But how?

One theory is that menstrually related migraines are triggered by falling levels of estrogen. But during pregnancy,
estrogen levels are consistently high. Some doctors believe
that the high levels themselves are therapeutic. Others believe
that it's not the absolute level of estrogen but its relative
constancy, the fact that it's not falling. Of course, neither
theory would explain why some women's headaches become
worse during pregnancy, even as most improve. Perhaps
rising levels of estrogen early in the pregnancy increase
headaches, but higher, stable levels do not.

Another theory for why women's headaches improve during
pregnancy points to endorphins, our body's natural defense
against pain. As we point out in chapter 2, endorphins are
remarkably similar to morphine in chemical composition and,
like morphine, produce a feeling of well-being, even euphoria.
Even women without migraine have reported a sense of ex-
traordinary well-being during the later months of pregnancy.
Perhaps the endorphins in some way counteract the migraineur's tendency to develop headache pain. (As has been
mentioned, endorphins are also produced by exercise, which
is why exercise is so highly recommended both for people with
headache and for those suffering from depression.)

A possibly related hypothesis concerns the role of *prostaglandins*. Whereas endorphins reduce our sensitivity to pain, prostaglandins heighten it. Prostaglandins may also be involved in triggering our blood vessels to constrict or dilate, actions that may be related to the cause of a migraine.

Higher levels of estrogen in the system stimulate the production of prostaglandins. Menstrually related migraine and dysmenorrhea (painful menstruation, cramping, etc.) seem to correlate to higher than usual levels of some prostaglandins and to lower than usual levels of others, including a prostaglandin known as PGI_2. During pregnancy, however, levels of PGI_2 tend to increase. These levels also increase when people with migraine take beta-blockers, a drug often used to prevent migraine. Thus, scientists hypothesize that the increased levels of PGI_2 during pregnancy help to prevent migraine as well.

Just looking at the levels of certain chemicals — prostaglandins, estrogen, and the like — or even looking at patterns of how the levels of these chemicals rise and fall, is probably not enough to truly explain the relationship of the female cycle to migraine, however. It seems that women who get only menstrually related headaches may react differently to prostaglandins during their menses. Why and how do they react differently? We don't yet know, although we suspect it has something to do with the complicated internal mechanisms that regulate a woman's "hormonal clock," determining which hormones are released in which combinations at which points in the cycle. In other words, like the complicated chains of biochemical events that intertwine to produce a migraine, the process of a woman's hormonal activity is both intricate and not yet very well understood.

Treatment of Migraine during Pregnancy

Naturally, developing drug-free ways of preventing and responding to migraine serves you well during pregnancy, when many drugs cannot be taken. Ergotamines, used to arrest headaches, are absolutely forbidden for pregnant women as they can abort the fetus. Most preventive medications should also be avoided.

Many of the substances migraineurs are encouraged to avoid — caffeine, alcohol, nicotine, foods high in processed sugar — are also off-limits for pregnant women. So the healthier diet recommended for pregnancy may have benefits for the prevention of migraine as well. Certainly regular aerobic exercise, relaxation techniques, biofeedback training, and attention to stress are useful both for coping with pregnancy and for dealing with migraine.

AFTER DELIVERY

Those women who enjoyed relief from headache during the second and third trimesters of pregnancy may find that their headaches have returned, with equal or greater force, after delivery. Some women even get their very first migraines at or soon after delivery. One study of forty women on a postnatal ward found that fifteen got headaches in the first week after giving birth, mostly within the first three to six days. Of course, women who had suffered from migraine before were more likely to get one at this time, but even some women who had never had migraines experienced their first one then.

Once again, the culprit seems to be estrogen withdrawal, the rapidly falling levels of estrogen that follow the end of pregnancy. One researcher suggests that falling levels of estradiol (a type of estrogen) makes the blood vessels more sensitive to the constrictive effects of serotonin, which in turn brings on the vasodilation that is experienced as a headache. (For more about how this process works, see Chapter 2.) However, only some women experience this sensitivity; we don't yet know why they do, and not others. It's also possible that pregnancy affects the metabolism of serotonin itself, in ways that in turn affect serotonin's role in producing migraine.

COPING WITH PREGNANCY AND MIGRAINE

As we repeat throughout this book, your biggest ally in your efforts to prevent and manage headache is your own awareness of your body and your own commitment to yourself. Pregnancy can be a wonderful occasion for learning anew how to listen to your body, become aware of your needs, and nurture yourself in effective ways. The benefits you derive from this approach to pregnancy will serve you well in your responses to migraine over the coming years.

As in pregnancy, a woman who is breast-feeding should be conservative when using any headache medication. However, drug levels in breast milk are 1 to 2 percent of the maternal blood level and some medications are insignificant to an infant's health. For instance, narcotics (e.g., codeine, morphine) and nonsteroidal anti-inflammatories (NSAIDs) are compatible with breast-feeding because only a small amount passes into breast milk. Acetaminophen and caffeine are also safe and are preferable to aspirin. A breast-feeding woman should avoid bromocriptine, sumatriptan, ergotamine, and lithium, and should use benzodiazepines, antidepressants, and neuroleptics with extreme caution. Aspirin is not recommended and should be used with caution. One way to decrease drug exposure to a nursing infant is to take medications just after completing a breast-feeding. If you must medicate, using a breast pump and saving the milk for a feeding may give your body enough time to eliminate the medicine.

CHAPTER 6

Menopause and Migraine

MENOPAUSE AND THE DOCTOR-PATIENT RELATIONSHIP

It's virtually impossible to speak about menopause without raising a host of emotional issues, as well as medical ones. In our society, where women are so often defined either in terms of their sexual attractiveness to men or in terms of their roles as mothers, menopause appears in many people's eyes to symbolize the end of both. Even if a woman herself does not accept this definition of her attractiveness, her sexuality, or her worth, she must often deal with the reactions of her family and friends, as well as with the negative images of "old women" that pervade the culture as a whole.

In addition to the psychological aspects of menopause, there are of course its biological effects, which are only imperfectly understood. This partial knowledge is to some extent because women's hormonal activity is extremely complicated in all its aspects, but also because menopause is just one of many "female problems" that have historically received all too little attention from the scientific and research establishments.

Thus, the relationship between menopause and migraine is a complicated one — for the woman herself; for her family, friends, and coworkers; and for her doctor or other health care provider. It's always important for headache-prone women to find doctors who take headache seriously as a valid biological disorder and to develop partnerships with their doctors based on mutual trust and respect. But such a physician and such a relationship are particularly important for menopausal women with migraine. At this time of her life, it's crucial that a woman work with a doctor who respects her, who treats her as a person rather than as a set of symptoms, and who encourages her to pay attention to her own physical and emotional responses as an essential part of her treatment.

Only you can really know which medications are working and which are not, which treatments suit your lifestyle and which do not. Treating migraine is already a complicated procedure that works differently in each individual case — but at least with migraine, you have had years to become familiar with your body and its reactions. Neither you nor your doctor has ever observed you going through menopause before, so a certain amount of patience and willingness to experiment with a variety of treatments must be present on both sides. Both of you must be willing to sort through the side effects of a new medication versus the hitherto unfamiliar effects of your particular place in the menopausal process. This sorting out is best done within the doctor-patient partnership that we describe in Chapter 2, in which both patient and healer take responsibility for the treatment and its success.

MIGRAINE AND MENOPAUSE: AN OVERVIEW

As might be expected, women with migraine react to menopause in a variety of ways. Most women seem to have more headaches as they enter and pass through menopause, with correspondingly fewer headaches afterward. However, there are a sizable number of women who respond otherwise at each stage of the process.

It's tempting to reason that since a woman's monthly cycle is implicated in menstrually related migraine, migraines should therefore disappear after menopause. In fact, although female hormonal activity is clearly involved in women's migraines, it isn't at all clear how the end of one part of that activity affects migraine. Both men and women tend to get fewer migraines as they get older, so clearly more than just women's biology must be involved. Perhaps the aging process and the process of menopause are two separate but related journeys, each with its own separate — and interacting — relationship to migraine. One theory suggests a decrease in serotonin receptors with age.

THE BIOLOGY OF MENOPAUSE

In our attempt to understand more clearly the relationship of migraine to menopause, let's look at the biology of menopause itself. As is described in Chapter 4, menstruating women undergo a monthly cycle in which a new ovarian follicle grows each month to release a new egg into the woman's fallopian tube and then womb. This process of releasing an egg is known as *ovulation*. Normal menopause (that is, menopause not caused by any organic problem or injury) results from the depletion of ovarian follicles that can be stimulated to release eggs.

Menopause is not a single event, but a process that may continue for several months or more. This process entails a number of biological changes, which vary throughout the body's process of getting used to its new condition.

Every woman past menarche (the start of menstruation) has an entire hormonal system set up to time the release of eggs, the nourishment of fertilized eggs (pregnancy), and the discharge of the womb's lining during the month when there are no fertilized eggs (menstruation). A number of body parts, including the hypothalamus, the pituitary, and the ovaries, are involved in releasing various combinations of hormones to facilitate this cycle, which affects a woman's metabolism, blood circulation, neurological system, and emotions.

When this system is no longer functioning, a woman's entire being is affected in a number of physical and emotional ways.

As menopause proceeds, female sex hormones like estrogen are at markedly lower levels than before, while other hormone levels rise. The hypothalamus — which houses the body's thermostat — behaves erratically, causing hot flashes and leading to surges of still other hormones. Hot flashes also correspond to new *vasomotor* activity, that is, the vascular system of arteries that carries blood throughout the body may contract and dilate in new ways, producing surges of blood (which cause hot flashes) and, possibly, triggering migraine.

Sometimes doctors treat menopausal women with estrogen replacement, using either estrogen alone or estrogen plus synthetic forms of progesterone. Many doctors claim that estrogen treatments bring women relief from the worst discomforts of menopause and reduce the chance of developing *osteoporosis,* a disease that makes the bones more porous and brittle — thereby putting postmenopausal women at greater risk of broken bones and other problems. Research also shows that estrogen replacement also reduces the incidence of repeat stroke in postmenopausal women who have had strokes.

Most estrogen replacements are given orally and cyclically, like birth control pills: twenty-one days on, seven days off. It is precisely this monthly cycle that seems to cause menstrually related migraine, so we recommend that migraineurs avoid cyclical estrogen replacement.

Doctors sometimes prescribe other additional hormones, including progesterone, intended to prevent endometrial cancer if the uterus has not been surgically removed, and androgens (male sex hormones), to treat decreased sexual drive and sexual responsiveness, fatigue, depression, and headache.

Estrogen treatments have generally proved controversial

because reportedly they themselves put women at increased risk of breast cancer. A 1992 review of this controversy in the *Journal of the American Medical Association* found no evidence for such risk among postmenopausal women, but the controversy continues to rage. When women need estrogen replacement, we recommend .05 mg daily doses of pure estradiol (by pill [Estrace, 1 mg] or patch [Estraderm]). If progesterone is needed, we recommend daily low doses of 2.5 mg.

HOW MENOPAUSE AFFECTS MIGRAINE

Since we know that estrogen and migraine are related in some way, it makes sense that menopause *would* affect migraine. What isn't clear is exactly *how* the two conditions interact. In many cases, it seems that falling and fluctuating levels of estrogen early on *during* menopause trigger migraines, just as falling levels of estrogen during the menstrual cycle seem to, at least in some women. Then, after menopause, when estrogen levels are low and stable, the body accustoms itself to those levels, and migraines — at least those triggered by estrogen activity — taper off dramatically.

This pattern is indeed the case for the majority of women, who start menopause by getting more headaches and end menopause by getting fewer. Some women, however, get more headaches during menopause, and some even get the first headaches of their lives at this time. We have yet to understand how the twin processes of menopause and aging affect these women.

It's also difficult to know what changes in exercise, diet, and lifestyle are prompted either by menopause or by aging — changes that may affect headache. For example, many women begin to contemplate their own retirement or that of a spouse at this age. They may also be dealing with their own or a spouse's age-related health problems or simply with a need to slow down. Women who have reached menopause may be watching their children grow up and leave home. Or their children may be getting married and producing grandchildren.

The emotional fallout from these problems will not necessarily be resolved as menopause is complete. The problems of retirement, failing health, and changing relationships with adult children may bring some women increased stress as they age, so that life after menopause contains more stress-related migraine triggers, perhaps with a corresponding decrease in the amount of time spent exercising. Increased migraines after menopause may indeed have a biological base but may also have an emotional foundation, or some combination of the two.

Likewise, menopause itself is an extremely emotional process for many women; certainly the consequent emotions — both those generated by the biological process and those inspired by one's thoughts and feelings about aging — may be a potent migraine trigger. Women without children are coming to terms with the fact that now they will never give birth to children of their own. Women who may have wanted more children are likewise coming to terms with the fact that this possibility no longer exists. Even women who are fully satisfied with their childbearing decisions may be deeply affected by the "official" ending of the more youthful portion of their lives. These issues are not necessarily resolved emotionally at the exact same time that the menopause process is resolved biologically.

MIGRAINE AND HORMONE TREATMENTS

Menopausal migraineurs may well be in a double bind: They may be suffering more from menopause than their non-headache-prone counterparts are, yet the estrogen replacement therapy that brings some relief to other women may be dangerous for them and may also be an additional migraine trigger, making the "cure" for menopausal migraine worse than the disease.

In our opinion, hormone treatments for menopausal women with migraine can be helpful in relieving symptoms such as hot flashes and mood changes and, if given properly, may not increase migraine.

It is true that in some studies estrogen replacement has even been shown to alleviate migraine. In other studies, it seems to exacerbate migraine.

If you and your doctor decide that, all things considered, hormone treatments are medically necessary after menopause, the purest synthetic estrogen may work better for you than one made from animal hormones. Also the lower the doses of estrogen, the better.

An estrogen skin patch (Estraderm), designed to release low, steady doses of estrogen into your system, is far less likely to cause the fluctuating levels of estrogen that seem to be related to migraine. The patch is placed on a piece of clean, dry skin on the abdomen or buttock and is changed twice weekly. It releases a steady amount of the naturally occurring ovarian hormone 17 beta-estradiol. Although no studies have yet confirmed the effectiveness of the patch in headache management of menopausal women, there is a lot of anecdotal evidence that it's a better form of estrogen treatment for migraineurs than cyclical tablets.

Other forms of estrogen replacement are available as a vaginal cream (Premarin, Estrace) or an injection. Estrogen implants are still in the experimental stage but seem to promise a steady release of the hormone similar to the estrogen patch. A new patch can be changed weekly.

HEADACHE MANAGEMENT FOR WOMEN TAKING ESTROGEN SUPPLEMENTS

If you and your doctor decide that estrogen replacement is the right treatment for you, and your headaches get worse, what can you do? One solution, of course, is to try reducing your dosage. Another possibility, as we suggest above, is to switch from animal-based estrogen to a synthetic brand, such as synthetic ethinyl estradiol, estradiol, or a pure estrone. However, one study found that ethinyl estradiol actually increased headache, whereas another type of estrogen, estropipate, taken orally, actually decreased the frequency and intensity of headache.

Another possibility is to stop taking oral estrogen and switch to a patch or, if available, an implant. Dr. Lee Kudrow, a noted headache researcher, reported a 58 percent improvement in headache control through reducing estrogen dosage and providing estrogen steadily (i.e., daily), rather than cyclically. In addition, for example, if a dose of Premarin is 0.625 mg once a day, better blood levels and fewer side effects may be achieved by giving 0.3 mg twice a day. Injections or vaginal creams may also prove better than pills. Some studies show that adding testosterone to the prescription also seems to help.

NONDRUG TREATMENT FOR MENOPAUSAL MIGRAINE

Although there is little we can say definitively about menopause and migraine, we can say that the type of body awareness we have advocated, along with the suggestions for diet and exercise in the following two chapters, can be invaluable for all women going through menopause, as well as for those with migraine. Avoiding alcohol, sugar, and salt probably helps both in preventing migraine and in reducing or alleviating menopausal symptoms. A vigorous exercise schedule (approved by your doctor) helps your body produce endorphins that both combat headache and ease the stress of menopause, creating a sense of serene well-being that helps you to weather the multitude of changes in your body.

For some women, menopause is a difficult time, either because of the biochemical changes it brings or because of the emotional and social changes it seems to symbolize. For other women, menopause is an easier passage. Many women have reported this time of life as the beginning of a new period of self-confidence and achievement. Relieved of their former responsibilities of caring for children, freed of their earlier preoccupation with the reactions of others, these women experienced menopause as heralding new opportunities for work, love, and self-awareness. "I no longer care what other people think about me," these women often say. "For the first time in my life, I'm free to live for myself and to do what I want — and it's a terrifying and thrilling possibility."

Whatever the process of menopause comes to mean for you, you'll be better able to make the most of this time if you don't also have to struggle with migraine. Working with your doctor and listening to your body helps you negotiate this major life passage.

CHAPTER 7

Diet and Nutrition for Headache Management

DIET: AN EMOTIONAL TOPIC

FOOD IS AN EMOTIONALLY CHARGED ISSUE for everyone in our society — and we've found that it is particularly so for women. Because of the pressure put on women to meet certain narrow standards of attractiveness, many women are preoccupied with gaining and losing weight. And because the literal role of cook and the emotional role of nurturer often fall to women, food as the symbol of love, caring, and comfort may be particularly potent for women. For women, as for all of us, food is often associated with powerful childhood memories, as well as with significant family occasions and important private rituals.

Because food's meaning in our lives is so profound, it's often hard for us to think rationally about what we eat and how it is affecting us. If having a warm, milky cup of coffee first thing in the morning is what gets you out of bed, you don't want to find out that it's giving you an addiction to caffeine that may be setting you up for a headache. If nibbling a piece of chocolate while watching your favorite TV program is your one reliable comfort after a long, miserable day, you certainly don't want to find out that it's giving you a migraine.

Yet often the foods that we love most and that we crave most intensely *are* headache triggers, at least under some circumstances. Often, too, the foods that we're most used to are affecting our bodies in painful or discomforting ways — but because we're so used to them, we just don't notice. Learning to consider the possibility that the treats and rituals that we grew up with are harmful to us — at least some of the time, to some extent — is never an easy lesson.

We believe that diet, as with every other aspect of headache, is an extremely individual matter. Each woman's response to food is unique and varies, depending on what else she's eating, how much exercise she's getting, what time of the month it is, and what emotional state she's in. Maybe that late-night chocolate doesn't trigger a migraine after a calm day but does so after a stressful day. And maybe if that stressful day is followed by a brisk aerobic workout, the chocolate has no effect at all. Maybe when you eat the chocolate on an empty stomach, it triggers a headache; whereas when you eat it with a glass of milk, a headache is averted — or maybe it always produces a headache.

Likewise, maybe that first cup (cups are fine — watch out for mugs!) of coffee is just fine — it's only when you follow it with a second cup in the afternoon that the caffeine may reach a headache-triggering level. Or you may find that you can give up coffee entirely, but you can't cut down: Once you start drinking it, you crave it more and more. Perhaps you can drink coffee during most of the month but not during the weeks just before and during your period. Or maybe once you give up coffee for a couple of weeks, you'll find yourself feeling so much better you won't *want* to go back to it, inconceivable as that seems now.

In the end, no matter how much information we or your doctors provide, the final decisions about your diet are up to you. We believe that the most important thing you can do is to learn to listen to your body, so that you yourself can realize what effects a food or beverage has on your health and well-being. Maybe you'll decide that the occasional late-night chocolate is worth a headache or two; maybe you'll take a chance on the coffee. But whatever you decide, you'll do so knowingly.

In this chapter, we explain an interesting theory that links migraine headaches to low blood sugar and offers a corresponding way of eating that has been dramatically effective in reducing headache. We let you know about the most common dietary headache triggers and tell you how to experiment to find out which foods, vitamins, and eating habits work best for you.

We start off with this suggestion: Take it one day at a time. Diet is extremely interactive. You may discover some foods to shun at all costs, but you might also discover ways to enjoy at least some of your favorite foods while still avoiding headaches. Perhaps exercise makes a difference; maybe you can have certain treats during the weeks you're not premenstrual or having your period; or you might find that once your diet as a whole becomes healthier, an occasional treat no longer has the same headache-triggering effect. If you allow yourself to view your diet as a *process* rather than as a fixed set of rules, you're well on your way to nourishing yourself in a way that brings you headache relief.

YOUR DIGESTIVE SYSTEM

To understand how "you are what you eat," let's begin where your diet begins — with the process of eating itself. When you take a bite of food, what happens?

As soon as food enters your mouth, the enzymes in your saliva start to break it down. When you swallow, the partially broken-down food passes through your esophagus, a long tube that leads into your stomach. The food breaks down further as your stomach releases chemicals of its own.

The next stop for your dinner is the small intestine, which completes the breakdown process. The food you've eaten now exists as its component parts: carbohydrates (a combination of carbon and water found in every living thing), protein, vitamins, minerals, fat, and waste.

All but the waste pass into your bloodstream through the wall of your small intestine. The blood carries these elements to the parts of the body that need them, so that the nutrients you've digested can fuel your energy and renew your bones, muscles, tissue, and nerves.

Anything that can't be used right away is stored, partly as body fat (which is how you gain weight) and partly as glycogen — a substance stored in the liver that can be converted into glucose, or blood sugar. Your body is always striving to keep your blood sugar at a certain level. Whenever the level falls too low — say, if your burn up glucose in vigorous exercise, emotional stress, or heavy thinking — the body draws on glycogen to make up the difference. If there is no available glycogen, you may feel light-headed, irritable, or worse. (For more about blood sugar and its effects, see below.)

Meanwhile, anything you can't use of what you swallowed is waste and passes into your large intestine. From there, it moves into your rectum, and is expelled.

Just as nutrients pass into the blood through the walls of the small intestine, toxins pass into the blood through the walls of the large intestine. The blood carries these toxins to the liver, whose job is to purify the blood so it can continue to nourish the rest of the body.

If your liver is not functioning normally it may not be able to do its job properly. Alcohol, nicotine, caffeine, recreational drugs, medications, hormones used to fatten cattle or poultry, preservatives, pesticides, spoiled foods, fatty foods, and rancid oil in snack foods are all experienced by the liver as toxins. If you're taking in too much of those "toxic" substances, there may be a strain on your liver.

As we noted in Chapters 4–6, your liver is interrelated with parts of your endocrine (hormonal) system. For example, it must break down any extra estrogen (female sex hormone) in your bloodstream, whether that estrogen is there naturally, as part of your menstrual cycle, or artificially, as part of a birth control pill or hormone-replacement therapy.

If your liver is working overtime, however, it may not be able to perform its functions properly, neither breaking down your estrogen, nor cleansing your blood of toxins, nor regulating the conversion of glycogen into glucose (blood sugar). The estrogens may remain in your bloodstream as a headache trigger. The toxins may do so as well. And your low blood sugar levels may constitute a third type of headache trigger.

Clearly eating in a way that is healthy is good for your liver and the rest of your body; it's your first step on the way to an antiheadache diet. Most Americans do not have a good diet but those of us with headache pay a special price for our disregard. You may know someone who can eat exactly as you do with impunity — but you are the one with the headache-prone system.

Being Good to Your Body

Many doctors believe that the following diet may lessen the frequency and intensity of your headaches. We can't offer much in the way of scientific data to back up these suggestions, since very little research has been done. And only you can decide how many of the following choices will work for you. However, you might want to see what happens if you experiment, possibly trying one new eating habit each week:

- only those medications that you and your doctor have agreed are absolutely essential
- juices, seltzer (particularly with low or no salt content), well or spring water instead of soda, including decaffeinated and artificially sweetened soda
- herb teas instead of caffeinated coffee, tea, or hot chocolate (cut out caffeine gradually, over a two-week period)
- relaxation methods instead of alcohol or drugs

- organic or homegrown vegetables instead of those sprayed with pesticides
- homemade snacks, nuts, seeds, or hot-air popcorn instead of prepared foods (you're particularly trying to avoid high fat, salt, and sugar content; food coloring; MSG; and other preservatives)

MIGRAINE AND YOUR BLOOD SUGAR

What is Hypoglycemia?

Let's go on to look at how the level of your blood sugar may be related to how often you get headaches. A potent headache trigger is *hypoglycemia,* or low blood sugar. Hypoglycemia is the opposite of *hyperglycemia* (high blood sugar), which is seen in diabetes. A diabetic's pancreas is unable to produce enough *insulin,* the hormone that enables the body to utilize glucose and also drives it into the cell. Hypoglycemics have the opposite problem. An overactive pancreas produces too much insulin, lowering their blood sugar too quickly.

Many doctors recognize only a strict definition of hypoglycemia, as measured by a person's blood sugar levels on a five-hour glucose tolerance test. We, however, believe that there may be less severe degrees of hypoglycemia, called *relative hypoglycemia.* This is a much milder form of the condition, which may produce any of the following symptoms:

- feeling anxious, irritable, depressed, extremely moody, or confused after missing a meal
- losing memory or concentration after a missed meal
- feeling dizzy, having tremors, or breaking into a cold sweat after a missed meal
- continually craving sugar or sweets, or finding that once you start eating sweets, you can't stop
- getting a headache after missing or delaying a meal

How Hypoglycemia Affects Your Body

In a healthy body, the cycle occurs smoothly: you eat, which drives your blood sugar up, triggering the release of insulin, which drives the blood sugar back down to normal. In a diabetic, the blood sugar level stays high, as long as three to four hours after eating or constantly, because not enough insulin was produced to enable the body to utilize the glucose. In a hypoglycemic, on the other hand, the blood sugar falls *below* normal, as the result of too much insulin.

Thus, if you're taking a glucose tolerance test for diabetes, a doctor can tell at the two-hour mark how your body has responded: either your blood sugar level is high (diabetes) or normal. If you're neither a hypoglycemic nor a diabetic, your blood sugar stays at a normal level for the next few hours.

If, however, you're a hypoglycemic, your blood sugar goes on to fall below normal between the second and the fifth hour after eating because your system has produced so much insulin that the blood sugar continues to fall far beyond the point that is comfortable for you. Consequently, if you are a hypoglycemic, you need to eat *something* every couple of hours, to keep your blood sugar level normal. (If you are being tested for the extreme form of hypoglycemia, make sure your doctor orders a five-hour test!)

Relative hypoglycemia may not show up in tests. But if the symptoms we've described sound familiar to you, read on. You may discover another way that diet can help you reduce and prevent headaches.

Headache and Hypoglycemia

Consider what happens when you eat a starch (pasta, bread, grains, potatoes) or a sugar (fruit, honey, processed sugar, corn syrup, or foods containing them). Your body breaks down the food you've ingested and turns it into glucose — blood sugar — that your blood carries throughout your body, along with oxygen.

Your brain, your heart, and every one of your organs and glands needs both glucose and oxygen in order to function. In fact, every part of your body needs those two substances, which is why free blood circulation is so important to your life and health. Because glucose is so crucial to your well-being — indeed, to your survival — its level is monitored by not one but several organs: your liver, pancreas, adrenal glands, thyroid, and pituitary. As needed, these organs all help to ensure that insulin is produced to lower high blood-sugar level. They also all help to produce symptoms that signal your body to eat more when you need to raise your blood sugar level.

When you eat; ingest processed sugar, caffeine, or alcohol; or use tobacco, marijuana, or cocaine, your blood sugar level goes up. This reaction is why cocaine, alcohol, caffeine, and nicotine tend to take away your appetite — your body is fooled by the increase in blood sugar into thinking that it's already eaten. Even marijuana dulls your appetite initially. (For the reason why it later makes you ravenously hungry, read on). Taking in food or any of those other substances alerts your pancreas to produce more insulin.

Insulin, in turn, enables the body to utilize glucose and helps glucose pass through your blood vessels into your body tissue, providing your body with the more or less continual nourishment that it needs. Cutting off circulation to any area of the body for any extended length of time could result in the "death" of that body area; it isn't receiving life-giving glucose and oxygen from the blood. This can cause a stroke, heart attack, gangrene, or other serious condition.

What happens if there's so much glucose in your blood that it can't all be absorbed by your tissues right away? The same insulin that helped the glucose pass through your blood vessels then "tells" your liver to convert the glucose to glycogen. When you need to raise your blood sugar level again — say, after more time has passed without eating, or after vigorous exercise has burned up some blood sugar — your liver converts the glycogen back to glucose, and your body is replenished again.

Of course, sooner or later, you have to eat. No one can survive on stored energy forever. But a healthy body can live on stored energy from glycogen for twenty-four hours after fasting begins before symptoms of starvation set in due to the breakdown of fat and protein.

The diabetic and the (relative) hypoglycemic can't negotiate this process so easily, however. After a healthy person eats, a normal pancreas lowers blood sugar down to 70 to 110 mg % (milligrams per 100 milliliters of blood). Insulin channels the rest of the blood sugar into the body's tissues. But a diabetic's pancreas can only shift enough blood sugar to get the level down to 130 to 300 mg %. Thus, a great deal of a diabetic's blood sugar isn't going where it's needed — unless the diabetic takes an oral blood-sugar-lowering medicine or injections of insulin. Otherwise, some sugar spills into the urine.

A hypoglycemic's pancreas, on the other hand, is overactive. It produces so much insulin in reaction to eating that the blood sugar level drops to 40 to 50 mg %. Too *much* glucose is leaving the blood vessels for the body's tissues. In relative hypoglycemia, the blood sugar level falls but remains in the low normal range. This can still produce symptoms of hypoglycemia in some individuals.

Why is this a problem? Only because your body experiences it as an emergency. It doesn't realize that the reason your blood sugar level is low is that the blood sugar has been channeled into the body's tissues, where, after all, it was needed in the first place. But your body only knows two states: safe (a normal level of blood sugar) and in danger (a low or falling level of blood sugar). Your body responds to its perceived state of danger by triggering one of our oldest survival mechanisms, the reaction of "fight or flight." In effect, your body is telling your brain, "This is an emergency! If we don't get more blood sugar soon, we may not be able to function."

Rationally speaking, your body is wrong. You just ate. (Or perhaps you just drank alcohol, ate a candy bar or other sweet food, or smoked tobacco or marijuana — all activities that can raise blood sugar levels very quickly, triggering a bigger-than-usual surge of insulin production and the consequent hypoglycemic reaction.) But biologically speaking, your body is *sure* that it is short of food, because it's reading the only meter it has: your blood sugar level.

What does the body do to get its glucose level back up again? It stimulates the adrenal glands, its way of coping with an emergency. One of the group of substances produced by your adrenals are *catecholamines* — chemicals in the form of neurotransmitters, like noradrenaline and serotonin. Noradrenaline's job is to constrict your blood vessels, so that blood travels through your body faster and with more force. Consequently, the little blood sugar that is left reaches all your body's tissues. If in fact you were starving, this would be a very useful reaction.

Catecholamines have several other effects as well, all of which are part of the "fight or flight" reaction to prepare you for an emergency: your body temperature rises (from the forcefully circulating blood) and has a direct effect on your thermostat in the hypothalamus; your blood pressure and pulse rate go up (to keep the blood moving); your breathing becomes shallower (so you can run or exert yourself in battle if need be); and you generally feel anxious, keyed up, alert, and ready for danger. Certain people may feel some of the symptoms described previously: a sense of panic, irritability, or despair (after all, you're facing a horrible emergency); difficulties with memory or concentration (how can you keep your mind on your work when you're in danger?!); and of course, a feeling of ravenous hunger (as far as your body knows, you're literally starving!).

Meanwhile, your constricted blood vessels can't stay clenched forever. Sooner or later, the opposite reaction must set in. Sure enough, the process triggers the release of another group of chemicals: the prostaglandins. As explained in Chapter 2, these chemicals dilate your blood vessels and produce inflammation, giving you that painful, throbbing headache that you may not realize you get after missing a meal.

Prostaglandins also sensitize your body to pain — a useful follow-up to "fight and flight." Although you wouldn't want to be too sensitive to pain *during* a fight or flight, you would certainly want a chance afterward to tend to any wounds incurred. In this case, the "wound" you've incurred is the headache itself, which the presence of prostaglandins may make even more painful.

As we've described this process, it sounds as though extra insulin leads directly to a migraine headache. However, this may be true only for people who are susceptible to migraine with that inborn biological predisposition to the effects of relative hypoglycemia to which we've referred. In one experiment, when migraineurs were given a shot of insulin, they reacted by developing a migraine. But when people without migraine were given a *double* dose of insulin, they stayed headache-free. And it's completely possible to be hypoglycemic and not get headache; only about half of all hypoglycemics do. So the process described is probably the result of yet another process, most likely having to do with noradrenaline, serotonin, and other neurotransmitters. In other words, like stress, menstruation, and the weather, hypoglycemia may be only a *trigger* of migraine headaches, not an ultimate cause.

It's also true that a missed meal can set off a headache at some times and not at others. Women notice that missed meals during their premenstrual or menstrual times may set off headaches, while at other times they can skip lunch with impunity. It may be that exercise; relaxation techniques; the resolution of certain emotional issues; a generally healthier diet; appropriate vitamin and mineral supplements; or cutting out caffeine, alcohol, nicotine, and similar substances may modify or even eliminate your tendency for relative hypoglycemia to produce a headache.

Eating Choices for Hypoglycemics

The best thing you can do if you think you've got relative (or more serious) hypoglycemia is to watch your intake of processed sugar, caffeine, alcohol, and other drugs. The specific effects of caffeine and alcohol are detailed later in this chapter.

Processed sugars are especially likely to trigger a hypoglycemic reaction because they have no other nutrients. If you eat, say, a brownie *and* a glass of milk, it takes your body a while to break down that snack into all its component parts — protein, fat, carbohydrate, and sugar. Only after this breakdown has begun does the sugar in the brownie make its way into your bloodstream.

If you eat just the brownie by itself, there's a lot more sugar and a lot less of the other ingredients. The sugar almost immediately makes its way into your bloodstream, sending blood sugar levels up in a "sugar rush" and triggering your pancreas to respond with a larger-than-normal dose of insulin. All that insulin makes your blood sugar go down extra fast — and the headache-triggering cycle has begun.

Thus, you can probably avoid a hypoglycemic reaction by avoiding processed sugar in the form of granulated and powdered sugar, honey, maple syrup, corn syrup, and dextrose. (Honey is especially deceptive, because bees are often fed processed sugar.) You should also avoid such sweet foods as cookies, cakes, ice cream, and candy. Think about eliminating or reducing the following foods: soft drinks, juices to which sugar has been added, canned or frozen fruit, baked beans, baked goods, dates, raisins, and dried fruits. Although certain other foods don't contain sugar, their high concentration of white processed flour is almost as bad, since it too converts very quickly to glucose; therefore, avoid pretzels and novelty snacks like Cheet•Os. While they don't contain white flour, potato chips do contain a high concentration of starch, unmitigated by other nutrients, so they convert quickly to glucose as well. In extreme cases, you may wish to avoid the many canned, frozen, and otherwise preserved foods that contain surprising amounts of "hidden" sweeteners, including "nonsweet" foods like canned soup and frozen vegetables. (Read labels carefully or avoid prepared foods altogether.)

If you're not willing to give up sugar completely, consider reducing its place in your diet. And never eat sweet foods on an empty stomach. This rule includes not drinking sweetened coffee first thing in the morning and not starting your day with a Danish or sweet roll.

The best approach is, if you must eat sweets, always to combine a sweet food with a food that contains protein. Starch and sugar are converted directly into glucose, while protein is converted into amino acids. So if you give your body two jobs to do — digesting protein *and* sugar — you slow the rate at which the sugar finds its way into your blood. You may be able to "fool" your pancreas into sending less insulin, thus avoiding both the sugar rush and the headachy crash.

Reading this section may immediately inspire you with the sense that since certain foods are bad for you, you'd like to cut them out. But what if you're having the opposite reaction? What do you do if you can't quite believe that sweet foods are triggering your headaches or that it will do you any good to cut them out?

We suggest that you give up sweets for a month, noting your reactions, and then add back items on the above list, one at a time, again noting your reactions. Thus, you can begin to see for yourself which items you can tolerate, which you can't, and what circumstances affect your tolerance.

Some of our colleagues advocate a strict diet of boiled

chicken or lamb, with boiled or baked potatoes or rice and distilled water as beverage, for those patients who believe diet is a factor. If there are no changes in headache frequency, it is doubtful that diet plays a role.

Eating Habits for Hypoglycemics

Generally, you should try to eat as regularly as possible, making sure that every couple of hours (if you're very sensitive) or every four to five hours (if you're less sensitive) you have some protein and a carbohydrate. The morning — after your long night without eating — is an especially important time to eat, preferably a whole grain bread or unsweetened cereal and perhaps some protein as well.

Some hypoglycemics need to eat a light snack, such as crackers and a mild cheese, just before going to bed, to keep their blood sugar levels up during the night. In extreme cases, hypoglycemics must set their alarms so that they can eat a few crackers during the night.

As you become aware of your body's warning signals, you can make sure to eat before the "panic attack" from lack of food (or from sweets) sets in. Some hypoglycemics carry emergency stores of cheese and crackers with them, just in case.

A healthy diet without sweetened foods would include lean meats, fish, and poultry; green leafy vegetables; cucumbers and squash; soybeans and related products, such as tofu and miso soup; fresh fruits in moderation (with a special effort to moderate citrus, which may trigger migraine); potatoes; and whole grains, including whole grain bread. Even white-flour products, such as pasta, include enough nutrients to make them relatively safe, however. A whole wheat carob cookie sweetened with honey is far more likely to trigger a reaction than plain old white-flour spaghetti.

As your diet and eating patterns change, you may notice that it's becoming easier for you to delay or even miss a meal. You may also learn to read when doing so is possible and when it isn't, depending on how much stress you're under or what time of the month it is.

Artificial Sweeteners

These won't trigger a hypoglycemic reaction but may be unhealthy for other reasons. Many studies suggest that saccharin may increase your risk of cancer, while aspartame (found in NutraSweet and Equal) seems to trigger swift and severe headaches in some people. The mechanism is unknown.

Generally, artificial sweeteners seem to increase people's craving for the real thing, and some studies have shown that they actually stimulate people to gain weight, because they interfere with the dieter's effort to change her or his metabolism through exercise and cutting back on fatty foods. In small doses, artificial sweeteners probably don't pose much of a risk, but in our opinion, you're better off without them.

FOODS THAT TRIGGER HEADACHES

Many people find that one or more of the following foods frequently trigger a headache: pork, game, and organ meats (including liver, sweetbreads, kidney, and brains); smoked and cured, aged, and packaged meat (including corned beef, cold cuts, salami, bologna, pepperoni, hot dogs, ham, bacon, and sausage); herring, caviar, and smoked fish; vinegar; pickled and fermented foods; aged cheese (such as cheddar, blue, Brie, and Gruyère); products high in yeasts (including doughnuts, coffee cakes, and breads — especially hot, fresh bread); chocolate; sugar and all products made with processed sugar or corn syrup; citrus fruits in large quantities; figs; cream; sour cream; yogurt; the pods of lima beans, navy beans, and peas; flavor enhancers such as monosodium glutamate (MSG); caffeine; and alcoholic beverages, especially red wine.

Dietary caffeine should be distinguished from medicinal caffeine. For acute headaches, the addition of caffeine to aspirin or aspirin plus acetaminophen enhances pain relief, requiring less analgesic. (In fact, Coca-Cola was invented as a treatment for "sick" headache by a pharmacist and may have been the first medicinal use of caffeine.) Overuse or abrupt discontinuation can trigger headache.

There are many ways that you might discover which of these foods are your own personal headache triggers:

- Follow your instincts. Sometimes, simply by asking yourself the question or by starting to pay attention to your memories and your reactions, it becomes clear to you what your "danger foods" are.

- Work with a nutritionist. Someone who really knows the subject of food may help you isolate which foods are problematic for your system.

- Try an elimination diet. Cut out of your diet all the above foods for one entire month. Then add one food back in large quantities every few days, noting its effect on you and your headaches. And if eliminating all of these foods for a month has *no* effect on your headaches, then food is not your problem and you certainly should be working with a doctor.

Cravings

Some cravings are your body's way of telling you what you need. But some are actually a sign of a deeper problem. One way to know if any food on the above list is a headache trigger is to ask yourself if you frequently crave it, particularly around the time you get your period or the week before. And if you stop craving a food after not having had it for a month, that's an excellent sign that the craving was not particularly healthy in the first place; you've stopped craving the food because you've gone through withdrawal and are now no longer "addicted" to it.

There are many theories about what food cravings actually are. One theory relies on the addiction model, especially with regard to coffee and sugar. Both substances give us a kind of rush. Your body grows to need that physical response, and you begin to crave the substance that produced it. The foods may be making you sick, but your body has trained itself to rely on them. Then, when you don't have those foods, you develop headaches in response.

Another theory suggests that the cravings are not the result of an addiction, but a symptom of the same biochemical disorder that produces our headaches in the first place. Somehow, the neurotransmitter problem also affects the hypothalamus, which regulates the body's appetite. In other words, the same problem produces the craving and the headache — particularly around a woman's menstrual period.

It's also possible that the factors indicated by each theory interact. Biochemical events in our brain may set up a craving for food, which in turn speeds up the headache process. Or a biochemical event sets up the precondition for a headache but does not trigger one — until you eat a "forbidden food," which is just enough to push you over the edge and into a headache. In other words, if you're on the verge of a headache anyway, following your craving for caffeine, sugar, or alcohol may ensure that you'll have head pain, whereas inducing yourself to have a few crackers and some mild cheese or other protein snack might actually reverse the headache process.

Allergies

Many people confuse the notion of *allergy* — when your body mistakenly reacts to a substance as though it were life-threatening, mobilizing its immune system in defense —

with *sensitivity,* when your body is overly responsive to the effects of a substance. If eating a piece of aged cheese sets off one of your headaches, for example, it's not because you're *allergic* to the cheese. It probably is that you're extremely *sensitive* to the tyramine in the cheese and that even a low level of this substance provokes a chemical reaction in your body. The difference is important because a sensitivity can be affected by a host of other factors, many of which you may be able to control.

Thus, many experts believe that allergies play a relatively small role in setting off headaches; it's *sensitivity,* in their opinion, that makes some foods headache triggers. Other researchers and nutritionists believe that many of us do have a number of minor, unnoticed allergies, which express themselves through headaches and other minor symptoms. Many *allergens* (substances that set off allergies) are found in foods that most people consider healthy — for example, wheat, corn, and dairy products — making it even harder to perceive them as the source of a problem. Some people are also allergic to grasses, pollen, mold, etc., and on occasion this can trigger a headache.

Certainly, each person's body is unique, and many people *do* have allergies to such foods as the following: shellfish, dairy products, eggs, corn, peanuts, wheat, rye, barley, citrus fruits, onions, vegetables in the nightshade family (tomatoes, potatoes, eggplant, and bell pepper), preservatives, additives and artificial coloring, tobacco, alcohol, chocolate, and sugar.

Let us repeat that most of the foods triggering headaches do so not because of allergies but because of the chemical reactions they trigger, reactions that headache-prone people are unusually sensitive to. The immune system — involved in true allergies — is not involved in these reactions; rather, the biochemicals of the brain are at the root of the problem. In any case, if you think you may have a food allergy that's involved in your headaches, or if you simply want to explore the role of food as a headache trigger, you may wish to work with a nutritionist. And, of course, if all other treatments have failed, it may be appropriate to consult an allergist; however, the yield in terms of headache relief is usually low.

HEADACHE TRIGGERS AND YOUR DIET

We've given you an overview of the types of foods, beverages, and other substances that can trigger a headache. Below is some more detail about the categories that different triggers fall into, along with an explanation of why they may trigger headache pain.

Amines

Your brain and blood vessels need amines to function. Yet these very substances also have the power to trigger a headache.

Some amines are manufactured within the body itself. These are known as *biogenic* amines. Other amines must be ingested through food or drink. Either can trigger a headache.

Biogenic amines seem to help regulate moods, blood pressure, heart rate, and sleeping patterns. Variations in amine levels seem to be related to various psychiatric and neurological disorders, including depression, schizophrenia, Parkinson's disease, and Huntington's disease. Amines also seem to be implicated in migraine. Indeed, people with migraine often seem prone to depression, and frequently families have a history of both, suggesting that these conditions may have similar biological bases (they may both reside on the same chromosome and be inherited together). Of course, depression might also be generated by frequent painful, uncontrollable headaches, but scientists suspect that it has a biochemical as well as an emotional etiology.

As we've already explained, some of the body's own amines may be involved in triggering headaches related to stress and blood sugar. When the body perceives that it's in danger of any kind, either from low blood-sugar levels or from an emotional stressor, it reacts by stimulating the adrenal glands, which in turn produce catecholamines, such as noradrenaline. These constrict the blood vessels and increase the heart rate to get the body moving for "fight or flight"— setting in motion the chain of events that ends in head pain.

It's also possible to ingest foods that contain amines. Although the body needs to take in amines to function, taking in too many seems to stimulate in migraineurs the same chain of events that triggers a headache: vasoconstriction, followed by the vasodilation and the release of prostaglandins that becomes a throbbing headache. (For more on how this process works, see Chapter 2.) Thus, foods rich in tyramine, such as red wine or aged cheese, may drive migraineurs' amine levels up to an unacceptably high level, setting the process in motion. Other foods rich in tyramine include pickled herring, liver, smoked fish, sour cream, yogurt, and yeast extracts.

Nitrites

This group of chemicals has been used since ancient Roman time to preserve meat. In our own time, some 12 billion pounds of nitrites are added to our food supply to prevent botulism, to give meat a special cured taste, and to turn it red or pink.

Nitrites also seem to trigger human blood vessels to dilate — a factor appreciated by patients taking prescribed nitroglycerin, which dilates their coronary arteries and reduces chest pain. For some people, however, this dilation can cause a dull, throbbing pain in both temples, usually within thirty minutes of eating the nitrite-treated food. This is the cause of the so-called *hot dog headache*.

Possibly, nitrites also combine with some amines to form nitrosamines, which in some animals seem to cause cancer. It's unclear what effect nitrosamines have on humans.

In any case, if you think you're susceptible to nitrite headaches, you should be aware that nitrites are generally found in the following foods: canned ham, corned beef, smoked fish, salami, bologna, sausage, pepperoni, summer sausage, bacon, and the all-American hot dog.

MSG

Monosodium glutamate (MSG) is often used in Chinese cooking and in American preserved foods to enhance flavor. The food enhancer Ac'cent is full of MSG, as are many other salt substitutes.

MSG is a component of protein and is chemically related to GABA (gamma-aminobutyric acid), another important neurotransmitter. Any substance that affects neurotransmitters is likely to be implicated in headache, and MSG is no exception.

MSG is chemically related to glutamate, an "excitatory neurotransmitter." It stimulates brain cells and may cause excessive electrical discharges. Some migraineurs are sensitive to it and develop headaches.

Many people react strongly to MSG, with symptoms such as sweating, anxiety, tightness and burning in the chest and stomach, flushing, mood changes, tingling in the hands, pain in the neck and eyes — and, of course, headache. An MSG headache is characterized by a sense of tightness, like a headband squeezing around the forehead; it is also felt as a pounding pain in the temples. It usually occurs within fifteen to twenty-five minutes after ingesting large quantities of MSG on an empty stomach; after meals that "camouflage" MSG within a wide range of other foods, the symptoms may be delayed or never occur.

Researchers believe that as many as 10 to 25 percent of the

population is sensitive to MSG. Nevertheless, twenty thousand tons of this substance are added to our food each year, in items such as TV dinners and microwavable frozen dinners; self-basting turkeys; foods in Chinese restaurants; instant gravy; processed meats; canned and dry soups; dry-roasted nuts; some potato chips; prepared tomato and barbecue sauces; salad dressings; tenderizers and seasonings, including Ac'cent and Lawry's Seasoned Salt; and weight-loss powders.

If you think you're sensitive to MSG, ask Chinese restaurants to prepare your meal without it. Avoid packaged and prepared foods, or read labels carefully: MSG may appear under the name of *hydrolyzed vegetable protein, hydrolyzed plant protein, natural flavor or flavoring,* and *kombu extract.*

Salt

No one knows why salt causes headaches, but it seems to be a type of trigger, especially in children. Possibly its role is to aggravate high blood pressure, which is often associated with migraine and other headache. Sea salt may be somewhat healthier than other forms. Salt is found in tamari and soy sauce, as well as in an astonishing number of packaged and prepared foods, including sweet foods. If you're interested in reducing the salt in your diet, it's not nearly enough to stop cooking with it. You have to cut down on virtually all foods that you don't prepare yourself.

Chocolate

This is nearly everybody's favorite food, which, legend has it, mimics the biochemical state of being in love. Certainly such a potent substance might be expected to have a powerful effect on the body's chemistry — and sad to say, it is one of the strongest headache triggers there is:

- The ground cacao seeds that make chocolate dark have a slight hypoglycemic effect.

- The sweeteners that make chocolate tasty have an even greater hypoglycemic effect.

- Chocolate contains caffeine, a third type of headache trigger (see below).

- This delicious treat also contains phenylethylamine, which, as an amine, constricts blood vessels, and so may also trigger a migraine.

Smoking

Leaving aside the other destructive effects of smoking, people who are prone to headache should be aware that nicotine is a vasoconstrictor. Your body can come to depend on this substance to keep its blood vessels constricted, so that when the effects of the nicotine wear off, your blood vessels dilate and throb in pain. As with all addictions, your body comes to need higher and higher levels of the outside substance to produce the same effect, so that even if you are a heavy smoker, your nicotine levels are continually falling below what your body needs to prevent a headache. (Consequently, people who quit smoking often suffer from headaches during the withdrawal period.)

Even if your involvement with nicotine hasn't gone so far as to give you "withdrawal headaches" between cigarettes, the vasoconstrictive effect of the nicotine makes your blood vessels unstable. This instability can make you more susceptible to headaches set off by other triggers.

Smoking also causes you to carry high levels of carbon monoxide and carboxyhemoglobin in your blood. These chemicals displace oxygen, meaning that your blood carries less oxygen to your brain. Your blood vessels react by dilating, in order to take in more of what little oxygen there is — and the result may be yet another headache.

Finally, smoking increases a migraineur's risk of cancer, hypertension, heart disease, emphysema, and stroke, particularly if the migraineur is also taking estrogen supplements in the form of birth control pills or hormone therapies. Such risks are increased because some migraineurs have spasms in the blood vessels that carry blood to their brains. Since smoking constricts these vessels, and since estrogen could cause spasms in the arteries, the migraineur who smokes and takes estrogen risks an arterial spasm in the vessels that lead to the brain. If the migraineur is being treated with ergotamine, an abortive medication that constricts the blood vessels still further, she may be putting herself in real danger. Postmenopausal women may gain some protection against stroke and heart attack from estrogen.

Caffeine

We don't tend to think of our morning cup of coffee or our afternoon tea as containing a powerful drug, but it does — caffeine. Caffeine may in some cases help relieve headaches, but by the same token it may also set them off. The stimulating effects of caffeine mirror many of the headache-triggering processes we have already examined.

Caffeine's lift comes from stimulating your adrenal glands, the part of the body that mobilizes you for an emergency. The adrenals produce noradrenaline, the substance that directs you toward "fight or flight." Noradrenaline production signals your liver to convert its stored-up glycogen into blood sugar, so you'll have more energy to cope with the emergency. If you've taken sugar in your coffee, tea, or soda, your blood is now getting blood sugar from two sources, the processed sugar and the converted glycogen.

This new high blood-sugar level stimulates your pancreas to produce more insulin. People who are hypoglycemic may react to this situation with extra-large surges of insulin. The insulin helps the blood sugar pass from your bloodstream into your body tissues — the sugar or caffeine rush. But once this process has been completed, your blood sugar levels are at a new low. Your body reads this low as a new emergency: not enough blood sugar. Your adrenal glands are stimulated once again.

Any time your adrenal glands go into action, your blood vessels are signaled to constrict, so that they can push the blood along faster through your body. After all, if you're going to fight or run away, you'll need this extra boost.

After the constriction, though, comes dilation. Now there's too much blood in your vessels, and you get a throbbing headache.

Most people don't get headaches while they're in the throes of the caffeine rush, because the caffeine is keeping their vessels constricted. When the caffeine wears off, however, their vessels may react violently, by dilating quickly, producing a headache. Consequently, many people wake up with a headache, which they "treat" by taking an early morning cup of coffee. The caffeine has worn off during the night, and they need a new infusion to constrict their arteries and get their blood moving again. Likewise, the phenomenon of "weekend headache" may be caused by caffeine withdrawal; when you sleep late, you're not getting your coffee at the usual time, and your body reacts by getting a headache. Also many people switch to decaffeinated coffee on the weekend, exaggerating the problem.

Of course, keeping yourself continually stimulated with caffeine might prevent headaches for a while, but eventually too high a level of caffeine produces headache. Also, as soon as you missed a cup at the usual time, you would probably react with a headache.

Keeping yourself continually stimulated with caffeine would require higher and higher doses. And as this dosage goes up, so do the caffeine's side effects.

The vasoconstrictive effect of caffeine is one reason why people who are prone to headache often turn to a strong cup or two of coffee when they feel the pain coming on. Sometimes, in fact, the caffeine can reverse the dilation of the blood vessels, constricting them sufficiently to prevent a headache. That's also why so many headache medications include caffeine (see chart below).

Caffeine in Your Diet

Source	Estimated Caffeine in Milligrams
Brewed coffee — one cup (five ounces)	100–150
Instant coffee — one cup	85–100
Decaffeinated coffee — one cup	2–4
Tea — one cup	30–40
Cocoa — one cup	10
Chocolate bar	25
Cola — 12 ounces	34
Anacin	32
Bromo Seltzer	32
Cope	32
Darvon Compound	32
Extra-Strength Exedrin	65
Midol	32
Vanquish	33
No Doz	100–200

However, using coffee to avert your headaches works best if you cut out caffeine from the rest of your diet. Thus, the caffeine you take at the beginning of a headache has an extra-powerful effect. (Some people prefer taking this pre-headache caffeine in the form of pills, such as Vivarin or No Doz rather than drinking one or two cups of coffee.)

If you think you may be getting headaches from caffeine

withdrawal, take a look at your coffee-, tea- and soda-drinking patterns. Do you drink more than two 5-ounce cups of American coffee a day? Then you're probably getting too much caffeine, although you may be so used to the drug's effects on your system that it *seems* to have no effect. Most people are susceptible to caffeine-withdrawal headaches with an intake of only 200 to 400 milligrams of caffeine (two to four brewed cups) a day, so take a look at the chart to see where your caffeine intake falls.

If you're prone to headaches and are taking in any caffeine at all, we suggest that you cut out all caffeine from your diet for an entire month. You may initially react by getting additional headaches, feeling drowsy and irritable, or experiencing other symptoms of withdrawal, but these should disappear within three weeks at most. If you're concerned about the symptoms, taper off gradually over the course of two or three weeks, cutting back by a half cup or a cup every four to five days. Then go for at least four weeks caffeine-free.

Many people who have given up caffeine — even those who previously derived enormous pleasure from it — report a new sense of well-being, much deeper and more restful sleep, an ability to get along better on less sleep, and an increased sense of energy. Some say that they were not aware of sleep or energy problems before cutting out caffeine, so they were especially surprised by the increase in their resources after they went caffeine-free.

If, after your experimental month, you still want to go back to caffeine, we recommend limiting yourself to one 5-ounce cup (not mug) of brewed American coffee per day, or its equivalent in other forms.

Decaffeinated Beverages

Unfortunately, even water-processed "decaf" contains chemicals used to remove caffeine from the coffee bean or tea leaf. Some of these chemicals have caused cancer in laboratory animals, although no studies have yet been completed on decaf's effect on people. We also know people who have reported feeling addicted to decaf, possibly responding to even the tiny amounts of caffeine that are left. Although these beverages do not usually trigger a headache, the final word on them is not yet in.

HEADACHES AND ALCOHOL

Although there's a lot of controversy over the relationship of diet to headache, the one substance everyone agrees is dangerous for headache-prone people is alcohol. Alcohol can cause headaches even in people who are not normally headache-prone, but it appears to be particularly potent for migraineurs and other people who regularly suffer from head pain. Red wine, sherry, and brandy in particular are virtually guaranteed to give most migraineurs a headache.

Alcohol and Your Body

Alcohol is such a potent headache trigger because it affects your system in so many different ways, each of which in some manner sets you up for a headache. To begin with, alcohol has a strong hypoglycemic effect; its high level of sugar and some of its other ingredients cue the pancreas to release insulin to combat the high level of sugar in the blood. The insulin, in turn, causes your blood sugar level to drop, and if you already have a tendency to hypoglycemia, this drop may trigger a headache. (See the section on hypoglycemia earlier in this chapter.)

In addition, many liquors contain tyramine and histamines, those amines that regulate, among other things, constriction of the blood vessels. A rise in the level of your body's amines may set off a corresponding reaction that ends in dilated blood vessels and a painful headache.

Alcohol also inhibits ADH (antidiuretic hormone), a hormone produced by the pituitary to help your body retain water. Drinking may then lead to increased urination and even dehydration. In longtime drinkers, these reactions become serious medical problems. Even after only one night of drinking, though, dehydration could give you a headache. Your brain floats in a pool of liquid spinal fluid, which keeps it stable and protects the brain within your skull. Alcohol-induced dehydration depletes spinal fluid, resulting in the pain of a hangover headache in many drinkers, whether they're headache-prone or not. Dehydration may also cause dehydration in the brain's nerve cells.

Other ingredients in alcoholic beverages are known as *congeners,* the impurities introduced during fermentation that give it its taste. Their presence varies according to the type of liquor or wine, but they are most prevalent in dark-colored beverages, such as red wine, brandy, scotch, and bourbon. Hence, if you must drink, avoid these and stick to white wine, gin, and vodka, preferably mixed with nonalcoholic substances, such as seltzer, orange juice, or tomato juice to increase the volume of water.

Finally, alcohol affects your liver in a variety of ways, all of which increase your vulnerability to headache. Chronic use causes cirrhosis, a serious liver complication.

To Drink or Not to Drink — And How?

Only you can decide which drinking patterns are right for you. Perhaps total abstention seems like the safest or easiest option, or perhaps it's important to you to work out a way whereby you can take a drink or a glass of wine at special dinners or at parties with your friends. Perhaps you can drink with impunity at some times of the month and not at others, or perhaps there are other ways of mitigating the effects of alcohol that allow you to drink in moderation and still stay headache-free. As we stress continually throughout this book, increased body awareness and the ability to read your own signals helps you decide what works best for you.

Meanwhile, here is some additional information that may help you make your decisions:

Some types of alcohol are more likely to provoke a hypoglycemic reaction than others. Sweet wines and liqueurs, of course, contain high amounts of sugar and affect you much as any sweet food might do. They only contain about 15 to 20 percent alcohol, but the combination of alcohol and sugar is a potent one.

That's because alcohol itself produces a hypoglycemic effect, even in drinks that don't contain any sugar. The most concentrated drinks — bourbon, brandy, cognac, gin, rye, scotch, vodka, and whiskey — each contain about 35 to 40 percent alcohol, and they signal your body to react by producing insulin.

Beer and ale might seem like a safe bet, since they have no sugar and only about 5 percent alcohol content. However, they are high in tyramine.

The safest alcoholic beverage for a headache-prone drinker is probably a dry white wine. It contains little or no sugar and only about 10 to 13 percent alcohol. Red wines, on the other hand, are rich in tyramine and congeners; they are highly likely to trigger a headache.

Drinking on an empty stomach has much the same effect as eating sweets when you're hungry: your body is hit with a rush of sugar or alcohol with no other "digestive work" to mitigate the effects. If before drinking you eat some protein and carbohydrates, along with a little fat, you help your body absorb the alcohol more slowly, with a less violent impact on your system. Of course, your ability to drive and your reflexes are affected in exactly the same way as always; you just won't *feel* so drunk. And you may be less likely to get a headache later. Drink a lot of water while you are drinking alcohol.

After a night of drinking, even if you've had only a glass or two of wine, drink several more glasses of water before you go to bed. You won't wake up dehydrated and headachy. Some people take vitamin C or even two aspirin or ibuprofen as well, to combat the effect of a hangover in advance. When you wake up the next morning, drink more water and some fruit juice; the water to combat dehydration, the fruit juice to raise your blood sugar levels gently. Do *not* drink more alcohol, as doing so will almost certainly make any headache worse.

DAIRY PRODUCTS

Dairy products include milk and any product made from it: cheese, yogurt, cream cheese, sour cream, and ice cream. Dairy products may be involved in headache because they cause you to produce increased amounts of phlegm and mucus, which block your sinuses. Although sinus problems usually don't cause your headaches, blocked sinuses may cause you additional discomfort during a headache. It's also possible that an allergy to dairy products triggers your headache pain.

Women, in particular, should be careful to get sufficient amounts of calcium in their diets, but it's possible to do so without relying on dairy products. Green leafy vegetables (kale, collards, chard, spinach, parsley, beet greens, and mustard greens), seaweed, nuts, grains, and, if necessary, supplements can provide you with all the calcium you need.

If you frequently feel that your head is clogged, or if you often feel your headaches in your sinus areas, you might try eliminating dairy products from your diet entirely for two to four weeks and noting the result. You may decide to eliminate them permanently, to cut down, or to avoid them at certain times: around your period, when the weather is damp and rainy (causing pain that you may also feel in your sinuses, along with the feeling of a clogged head), or at times of particular stress.

VITAMINS: HEADACHE RELIEF OR HEADACHE TRIGGER?

If you've been searching for a nutritional approach to relieve your headache, you've probably run into a lot of contradictory information about vitamins. Will more vitamin supplements help you prevent headache? What about the so-called megadoses of vitamins — are they safe? Are they effective? Does a person who eats a healthy, well-balanced diet really need to take vitamin supplements?

We believe that in theory, a healthy diet *should* contain all the vitamins and nutrients that a person needs. However, in our society, many fresh fruits and vegetables reach us depleted of vitamins by the way they've been shipped or stored. Furthermore, stress, alcohol, and caffeine all tend to deplete our body's supply of B vitamins, so many people experience shortages of those essential vitamins. Finally, a busy life may mean that it's not always possible to eat enough of the right kinds of foods all the time to ensure a constant supply of necessary vitamins. Therefore, vitamin supplements may be helpful, both to address all-around diet issues and specifically to help combat headache.

B Vitamins

The most helpful vitamins for people with headache are the B vitamins. In fact, headache-prone people may actually be suffering from a lifelong deficiency of them. They help the body cope with stress and aid the *intermediary metabolism*, the molecular transformation of food into substances that the body can use. People with hypoglycemic tendencies may benefit from the role of B vitamins in metabolizing sugar and carbohydrates.

Niacin

One of the B vitamins, niacin has a direct impact on the circulatory system: it dilates the blood vessels. If you are feeling tense and stressed-out, you may feel your blood vessels constricting in an effort to help meet your emergency. Taking 50 mg of niacin can dilate your blood vessels, helping you to calm down and also preventing a *later* dilation of blood vessels that might cause a serious headache.

Niacin often produces the so-called niacin flush, in which the dilated blood vessels cause a person's skin to itch and feel hot, perhaps turning red or blotchy. If you take niacin while your vessels are constricted, you may help avert a headache; however, some people get a headache from the dilation brought on by the niacin *so be careful.*

Vitamin B_6

We actually suggest that our headache patients take an extra 50–100 mg of this vitamin each day, with a higher dosage around the premenstrual week. More than 200 mg per day, however, can bring on nerve dysfunction. Natural sources of B_6 include broccoli, green peas, potatoes, tomato juice, beef, chicken, and ham.

Vitamin B_2

Recently it has been shown that large doses of vitamin B_2 (riboflavin) can help decrease migraine. It stimulates energy production in the mitochondria, or power pack, of the cell. We start patients at 100 mg per day. The proper dose is not yet known. Some studies suggest a gradual increase to 400 mg per day.

Vitamin A

Vitamin A supplements in the proper doses can relieve problems in the sinuses, as well as benefit your skin, eyes, and overall sense of well-being. High doses of vitamin A, however, can trigger headaches in headache-prone people, while non-migraineurs might develop *pseudotumor cerebri,* a serious illness characterized by headaches, double vision, and increased pressure on the brain. People who have been prescribed tetracycline (a common acne medication) can also develop pseudotumor, so they should be particularly cautious about taking vitamin A also.

COMING TO TERMS WITH DIET

One of the most frustrating aspects of being prone to headache is having to face the fact that our body limits what we are able to do. We'd like to be able to stay out all night drinking, to eat chocolate when we crave it, to enjoy a steaming cup of coffee when we're in the mood for its comforting warmth and reassuring lift. Sometimes we'd like to drop in to a fast-food joint with our colleagues from work, pick up a snack from the candy machine downstairs, or eat some of everything at the table at our family Thanksgiving feast. But if we know that a headache will follow, it can feel like a terrible, unfair punishment. "Everyone *else* gets to eat Dad's special ham salad — why can't I? . . . Everyone *else* in the office is going out for a pizza — but cheese *and* pepperoni *and* oil? I just couldn't!"

For women who may already have felt that they were perpetually on a weight-loss or weight-maintenance diet, the added burden of becoming aware of headache triggers might seem like the last straw. If a woman feels that she's already counting every calorie that goes into her mouth, watching out for tyramine and hypoglycemic effects may seem like more than she can bear. And, of course, if a person has counted on drinking caffeine or smoking cigarettes to help keep her weight down, forgoing the appetite-suppressing qualities of these substances may look like an impossible task.

All we can say is that knowledge is power. If you can turn the situation around from feeling victimized by this new information to *feeling empowered* by it, you can start to feel like you're making food choices that really do satisfy you. Maybe there's a way you can keep some of your favorite foods in your diet by committing to exercise, by cutting out alcohol, or by watching what you eat and in which combinations. Maybe you'll find that there are some foods you genuinely don't miss after trying life without them for a month or so. Maybe some food or alcohol treats will still seem so pleasurable that you're willing to risk an occasional headache in order to enjoy them.

Whatever you do, find a way to put yourself at the center of your diet decisions. The information in this chapter is meant to help you make choices, not to force you into restrictions that aren't comfortable for you. The reality may be that certain foods set off headaches in the biochemical system that you happened to be born with. But how you deal with that reality is up to you.

CHAPTER 8

Emotional Outlets: Understanding Stress and Learning to Relax

WHAT IS STRESS?: A MIND-BODY APPROACH

WESTERN SOCIETY TENDS TO DISTINGUISH between the mind and the body, but the latest biochemical and anatomical research suggests that this may be a false distinction. Virtually every emotional state that a human experiences has its corresponding physical event within the brain. Biochemical events can affect moods, thoughts, and perceptions; feelings and attitudes can affect a person's biochemical and physical state.

How does this apply to headache? We've already seen that emotions don't *cause* headache. A biochemical predisposition does that. However, a person with that biochemical predisposition may *translate* stress into headache, just as a person born with a predisposition to diabetes (and being treated with insulin) may translate stress into insulin shock.

The word *stress* itself has become a very loaded term, carrying the connotations of "overwork" and "emotionally worn out." In fact, the term — which is technically "stressor" — really means only "a demand to which the body must respond." Feeling slightly cold is a stressor, to which most people respond by going to get a sweater, turning up the heat, or refocusing their concentration to ignore the cold.

Feeling excited about seeing the person you love is a stressor; so is being given a surprise birthday party, being the honored speaker at your alma mater, or racing downhill on your favorite ski slope. All these pleasurable events place demands on our systems, causing us to mobilize our physical and emotional resources.

To some degree, although our minds can tell the difference between stress from (emotional) pleasure and stress from (emotional) pain, our bodies can't. On one level, our physical responses don't distinguish between the happy events just described and, say, being called into your boss's office, preparing dinner for your unpleasant in-laws, or having to prepare a fifty-page report in only six short hours.

Thus, people who get headaches on weekends or vacations may truly say that they love their jobs, that they find the demands exhilarating and exciting, that they genuinely enjoy the challenge, even though their doctors may point out that "letdown" headaches — *after* the stress is over — are a common response to on-the-job tension. If you too insist that your beloved, demanding job couldn't possibly be causing your headaches, you're not necessarily in denial. But, since you were born with a predisposition to headache, you may need to monitor your physical responses to even exciting and pleasurable challenges, finding ways to diffuse or alter their effect on your body, even as you continue to enjoy them mentally and emotionally.

It may also be true that you *don't* enjoy all the stressors in your life. Perhaps you feel you have to spend too much time being nice to people you don't really like, to do work that is boring or demeaning, to continually put others' needs before your own. Perhaps you love what you're doing *most* of the time, but you long for more time to relax. Perhaps you have mixed or confused feelings: you love your significant other, but the two of you are always fighting; your kids are your joy, but you just feel so drained; you wouldn't give up your job for anything, but you'd cheerfully strangle your boss and two of your coworkers.

Headaches are only a signal that *something* in the mind-body relationship may not be working properly. They don't really tell you what's wrong or why; that's something only you can discover. The suggestions in this chapter range from simple relaxation techniques that require only a slight increase in body awareness to psychoanalytic counseling that involves asking basic questions about your life. Taking one approach neither requires nor precludes taking another.

You may find, in fact, that the more successful one approach is, the more enthusiastically you are drawn to explore further. Or you may decide that since relaxation techniques are working for you, you really don't need to do any deep psychological probing. If you're also looking at issues discussed in Chapter 7 on diet, you may feel that you need to take things one step at a time — for example, first changing your diet, then developing a regular pattern of aerobic exercise, and finally learning how to apply relaxation techniques. On the other hand, approaching things physically and/or psychologically may mean that you can keep eating more of your favorite foods.

This chapter is intended as a grab bag of suggestions for ways you can help yourself ease the physical and emotional effects of stress in your life, with the ultimate goal of removing or reducing stress as a trigger for headaches. Maybe your headaches are a signal that deep down, you want to make some big life changes; maybe they're just telling you to breathe more deeply once in a while. One thing's for sure: They are *not* telling you that you are a bad person, that you enjoy making yourself sick, or that you have a "migraine personality." With that message firmly in mind, we invite you to explore some new aspects of the mind-body relationship as it relates to headache.

STRESS AND RELAXATION: YOUR BODY'S RESPONSES

Did you know that the stress response is automatic, but the relaxation response is not? Therefore, when your body feels itself to be in danger — whether that perceived danger is coming from a physical threat, an emotional issue, or the anticipation or memory of an emotional issue — it automatically goes into "brace position": shoulders hunched as if to protect your head; muscles tight in preparation for "fight or flight"; constricted blood vessels to fuel those ready muscles; rapid heartbeat and quick, shallow breathing to further support the body's rapid response to danger.

This response is so automatic, many of us are not even aware that we have it. In fact, those of us who lead busy, demanding lives may think that being physically keyed up *is* our normal state of relaxation!

Right now, as you're reading this, run a quick check over your body. Are your breaths coming from deep down in your diaphragm (put a hand on your stomach to check), or from high up in your chest? What happens when you consciously allow a breath to fall all the way down to your diaphragm, on a slow count of four, and then gently release it through your mouth, on another count of four? Is it hard for you to slow down your breathing this way? That difficulty may be a signal that you are carrying tension, even as you're reading this book.

What about your muscles? Can you allow your head to drop, loosely, so that your chin touches your chest? Do you feel a strain at the back of your neck when you do that? Perhaps you're carrying tension in your neck. What about your lower back — can you feel any tightness in the muscles down there? Where are your shoulders — dropped and relaxed, or slightly hunched and thrust forward?

Put your hand on your heart and feel it beating. Then try taking ten deep breaths, in and out each on a slow count of four. (If the very *idea* of doing this makes you impatient, that may be another sign of the fast tempo at which you live your life.) Then put your hand on your heart again. Can you feel the difference?

As we point out, many elements of the stress response can trigger a headache. In Chapter 7 we describe in detail the body's response to a perceived emergency, including the adrenal gland's tendency to secrete certain hormones that in turn stimulate the pancreas to secrete insulin. This is a very useful response to an emergency, especially a primitive "fight or flight" emergency: the insulin helps make more blood sugar available to us, so that our muscles can use it for energy.

If you have tendencies to hypoglycemia — as many headache-prone people do — the lower or falling blood-sugar level becomes an emergency of its own. Your pancreas has released so much insulin that your blood sugar level falls way below normal, perhaps making you confused, irritable, unable to concentrate, anxious, depressed — even prone to cry or to fall into uncontrollable fits of temper. These reactions increase your body's sense of danger and thus increase your stress.

In addition, your hormonal reactions to this condition may set off a chain of biochemical events that results in a headache. (For more detail on headache and hypoglycemia, see Chapter 7.) Even if you don't have hypoglycemic tendencies, your muscles may contract or your blood vessels constrict as part of the stress response, laying the ground for a migraine, tension-type, or mixed headache.

You can interrupt this process in two different ways:

- *You can perceive this stressor differently and so react differently to it.* In other words, something you once considered an emergency you now consider par for the course. Something that once made you furious you now accept calmly. Something that once deeply distressed you,

you now find funny or interesting. (Some people find it helpful to get counseling as part of making these perceptual changes.)

- *You can perceive the stressor in exactly the same way but modify your physical reaction to it.* That jerk in accounting still makes you furious — but now you relax your muscles and breathe deeply after the first spurt of anger has passed. That eleventh-hour deadline still thrills and excites you, but now you run a quick check to make sure you're not holding all of the excitement in your lower back. That week of fighting with your teenage daughter is just as distressing as ever, but at the end of every day you blow off the tension with a brisk walk around the park and a soothing hot bath afterward. (For more about these responses to stress, take a look at the next few sections.)

Relaxation: A Way to Prevent Headache

Why are relaxation techniques so effective in interrupting the headache process? Because relaxation slows down the sympathetic nervous system, which constitutes one-half of the autonomic nervous system. That system in turn is the part of our brain that controls the "automatic" functions of our body: breathing, heart rate, the size of our blood vessels, the level of our blood pressure, the production of sweat, and the size of our pupils.

The sympathetic nervous system also regulates sleep, as well as feelings of alertness and relaxation. Therefore, slowing down this system not only interrupts many of the processes that lead to headache but also creates a feeling of calm and well-being, while the relaxed person remains alert and available to others' or her own needs.

Another beneficial aspect of relaxation has to do with breathing. Even though a relaxed person takes fewer breaths per minute, those breaths are deeper and fuller, bringing more oxygen into the lungs and, from there, into the blood. As noted in Chapter 2, when not enough oxygen is available to the brain at high altitudes, the blood vessels leading to the brain tend to dilate: they're trying to get as much blood as possible, so that they'll receive more oxygen as well. When deep breathing sends more oxygen into the brain, there's no need for those blood vessels to dilate; consequently, there is less chance of a headache.

Stress releases noradrenaline and other *catecholamines,* neutrotransmitters that seem to stimulate headache in some people. Relaxation, on the other hand, lowers the catecholamines in the blood.

RELAXATION TECHNIQUES

In this section we offer you a variety of relaxation techniques that you can do on your own. Some can be done in the course of a busy day; others require putting aside half an hour or more of "quiet time." If just the *idea* of finding half an hour a day to relax makes you nervous or angry, we especially urge you to try it, just for a week, just as an experiment. You may find that the decision to give yourself this time is even more beneficial than the relaxation itself.

Deep Breathing

Deep breathing helps you "bring yourself down" into a state of calm, relaxed concentration whenever you choose. Dancers, actors, and other performers use these techniques all the time to translate their stage fright into a sustained and focused performance. You can do the same.

First, practice breathing in through your nose, out through your mouth. Your nose hairs, or *cilia,* help purify the air that you breathe in, and air that comes in through the nose seems to go straight into the brain.

Next, put your hand on your diaphragm — the area just below your ribs, where your stomach is. When you breathe, you should feel yourself filling up with air. Your diaphragm should puff out, your chest should expand, and you should feel the air going way down below your chest. *Never* suck in your stomach or diaphragm while breathing in; always puff out.

If you're having trouble feeling breath expanding your diaphragm, lie on the floor on your back and place your hand on your stomach. Feel the air falling in and floating out. Now that you've felt this sensation, you can duplicate it any time you want to, even when you're sitting upright at your desk or standing in front of a crowded meeting.

Once you can feel the *deepness* of breathing, help yourself to slow down. Breathe in to a slow count of four, hold your breath for four counts, and breathe out to the same count. When you have mastered this, up the count to six, then eight, then ten, and finally twelve. Let yourself do it effortlessly, the air falling and floating rather than being sucked or pushed. Keep your exhales, in particular, slow and even, the same amount of air leaving you on each count.

Some people like to add an image of breathing in something good, like love or calm or peace, and breathing out something bad, like tension or anger or worry. Other people like to allow the breathing to empty their minds, concentrating only on the bodily sensations.

A great technique for calming yourself down is to slow down your breathing: breathe out on a count of four, then five, then six, on up to twelve. This exercise is great to do in a car, on public transportation, or while waiting in a public place. You can't *do* anything to speed things up, so why not allow yourself to slow down?

Many doctors feel that five minutes of deep breathing leaves you feeling as relaxed and refreshed as an hour's nap because the oxygen refreshes your brain cells. You don't have to set aside five whole minutes for deep breathing to work, however. You might check in with yourself any time you think of it, and remind yourself to breathe deeply. You might turn to deep breathing when you're aware of feeling tense, anxious, or upset. You might find times when you can't do anything else anyway — such as when you're stuck in traffic or on hold on the phone — so take five minutes out to breathe deeply then.

If you find yourself especially resistant to breaking the flow of work in order to take a relaxation/breathing break, you might ask yourself why this seems so difficult. Perhaps you could commit to an experiment: take two 5-minute relaxation breaks a day and then evaluate the experience at the end of the week. All in all, were you more or less productive?

Progressive Relaxation

The first time you try this technique, allow yourself a good fifteen minutes at least; half an hour is better. Your goal is to allow yourself to feel completely relaxed so that when you find yourself feeling tense in the middle of your daily life, you can recover the feeling of complete relaxation.

Lie down on your back, either on a firm mattress or on a comfortable floor. Some people like a pillow beneath their heads or their knees.

Allow your breathing to become deep and even, perhaps slowing yourself down on a count. Then inhale, hold your breath, stiffen one arm, and lift it. Clench it as tightly as you can, then exhale slowly, relaxing the arm and letting it drop. Repeat this process with each part of your body: the other arm, each leg, your abdomen, your shoulders and upper back, and your face. Then say to yourself, "I am completely relaxed and I feel wonderful." Allow yourself to remember a word, an image, or a sensory detail from the experience so you can bring back the total relaxation whenever you want to.

Overall Body Relaxation

This exercise, which takes about ten minutes, can be done either at the end of a stressful day or while you are actually having (or getting) a headache.

Lie down in the comfortable position described above, perhaps dimming the lights and loosening your clothes. Begin and continue the deep breathing you've learned. Linger on every part of your body, allowing it to relax. Start with your toes, then your heels, then your ankles, calves, thighs, buttocks. Relax your abdomen, chest, the base of your spine, the middle of your back, upper back, shoulders. Feel the relaxation moving through your upper arms, elbows, hands, and each finger. Feel the relaxation in your neck, chin, jaw, face, eyes, forehead.

Some people enjoy "telling" their tension to go away. Others use imagery, seeing tension depart in a puff of smoke or flow out of them like water. Keep breathing deeply and enjoy the sensation of cleansing oxygen moving through your body.

When you are completely relaxed, say to yourself, "It's safe to let go." Enjoy the sensation of complete relaxation. Then stretch and sit up very slowly. Enjoy the sensation of being relaxed and alert. Allow that sensation to stay with you as your continue on your day.

If you like, make yourself a relaxation tape with your voice or a friend's commanding you to relax each part of your body, perhaps with soothing music in the background. Be sure the speaker pauses five to ten seconds before naming another body part.

USING YOUR MIND TO HEAL YOURSELF

Your mind can be a powerful ally in relieving you of headache pain. These techniques help you enlist your mind's ability to create images, to analyze and explore, and to direct your thinking in positive ways.

Autogenic Training

Another term for this technique is "self-hypnosis." It's a way of talking yourself into a relaxed and positive state. Your goal is to feel warm (so that the blood vessels away from your head are fully dilated, stabilizing the vessels around your head to counteract migraine) and heavy (so that your muscles are fully relaxed, to counteract tension-type headaches). You can also use this technique either to prevent or to respond to a headache.

You'll probably want to learn this exercise while isolating yourself and lying down. Once you're familiar with it, though, you can do it in any relatively private place, even while sitting up.

Lie on your back in the position described above and begin your deep breathing. When you're ready, make suggestions to yourself in a positive mode, in the present tense, for example, "My right arm is warm and heavy. My left arm is warm and heavy. My right leg is warm and heavy. . . ." and so on. Continue through your abdomen, chest, back, and shoulders. Then tell yourself that your heartbeat is slow and powerful, your breathing is deep and cleansing. Finally, tell yourself that your neck and head are heavy and cool — heavy because relaxed, cool because there is no excess blood there.

If you use a negative suggestion —"My arm is not tense"— you'll find that your subconscious hears only the negative word, ignoring the "not." Always make positive statements in the present tense. Also, be sure to repeat each suggestion as often as you need to. You may want to move on from a tense part of the body to a more relaxed part, then come back to the first part later. Sometimes it takes a few tries before you can make the exercise work for you.

At the end of the exercise, say to yourself, "I feel completely relaxed and refreshed." Pause, enjoy that feeling, then stretch and get up slowly.

Why does this exercise work if it isn't really "true"? Well, somehow, by saying that you *are* relaxed, you make yourself relaxed, just as by saying that a placebo is going to cure you, sometimes you cure yourself. If you feel skeptical, allow yourself to suspend your disbelief for a week — and try this technique every day. Did it help your headaches anyway? If not, you can always try something else! You may be surprised, though, at the power of your mind to affect your body.

Creative Imagery

You can use this technique after a relaxation exercise or while you are actually having a headache. In either case, the technique is good both for improving your physical and mental outlook and for learning something about yourself and your headaches.

Find a relaxed position and breathe deeply and slowly. If you feel yourself getting tense at any point, go back to your breathing and calm yourself down.

Then allow your mind to create images that bring you relief from headache. Here are some suggestions for different approaches. Try these — one at a time is probably best — or create your own approach.

Visualize yourself lying in a cool stream and feel the water washing away your tension or your headache. See yourself wandering down a shady path in the woods and meeting someone you completely trust and love, who gives you a magic potion that instantly cures your headache. Imagine yourself surrounded by a pure white light that makes you feel comforted and safe; as the white light flows through you, your headache lifts and dissolves. Picture a light that grows until it is a bright, pulsating mass; then it shrinks and disappears. Now picture the same thing happening to your headache. Picture breathing your headache out into a cloud;

see it leaving you with each breath; imagine the cloud's color, texture, smell, and any other details you can picture; then imagine changing the cloud into a beautiful scene or object and breathing it back into your head.

Another type of approach is to visualize your headache: as a murky shape, a wild animal, a blazing fire, or a bolt of lightning. Allow yourself to identify details of taste, smell, texture, temperature, color, and sound. See if you can simply observe this image, as though it were quite separate from you, as though your only task were to gather information.

Then allow yourself to change the image into something gentle, healthful, or kind. Some people like to ask the image itself for permission to change it. Others enjoy the sense of mastery that transforming it gives them. If the image is a clawing beast, you might transform it into a tame and loving kitten, picturing yourself feeding and stroking it. If the image is a jagged, fiery red, see it transform into a cool, watery blue. Allow yourself to picture as much sensory detail as possible.

Some people like to send their final images away; others like to keep them. Either way, when you are ready, return from your focus on the image to a new focus on your own body. Revisit each of your limbs, your chest, your back. If there is tension anywhere, breathe it out. In any case, keep breathing deeply. Stretch and get up slowly.

Yet another alternative is to ask your headache questions after you have visualized it. Why is it here? What does it want? Does it have a message for you? Ask it what you can do to ease the pain, how you can prevent the pain. Allow your mind to wander freely through these questions and answers, without judging or evaluating, simply allowing whatever words or images that emerge to float through your mind. Let yourself notice and remember them. When you're ready, tell your headache that you heard what it said and then respectfully ask it to leave. Return to an awareness of your body, perhaps again going through progressive relaxation. Then stretch and sit up slowly.

After any of these exercises, you may find it useful to write in a journal, recalling what you've experienced and adding other feelings, associations, memories, or insights that emerge. If you find this type of writing helpful, you may wish to do the same thing with your nightly dreams. The idea is that you may be using your headache to tell yourself something. If you can hear the message in another way, you may not need to suffer the head pain.

Another way to use creative visualization is to picture yourself in a real-life situation that you find difficult, such as hurrying to meet a deadline, fighting with a mate, or being tempted by a glass of wine that you know will trigger a headache. Picture the situation in as much sensory detail as you can: What do you see, hear, smell, taste, feel? What feelings and thoughts come up as you visualize it?

Then picture yourself responding in a new and satisfying way: You take a ten-minute break and yet you make the deadline anyway; you laugh the fight away or talk things out assertively and calmly; you see yourself turning away from the wine and drinking a delicious glass of iced apple juice with a cinnamon stick and cloves. The theory is that if you can visualize yourself behaving as you would like to, your real-life behavior will soon follow!

Affirmations

These are similar to autogenic suggestion, but you don't need to be in a deeply relaxed state for them to work. Find a list of positive statements that you want to make about yourself and practice saying them silently at frequent opportunities.

Some affirmations that people have found helpful are "I am calm and relaxed, and I have time for everything," "I love myself and I am loved," "I am a valuable person and I contribute a lot to the people in my life," and so on. As with autogenic statements, always be positive: Saying "I'm not really a bad person" will make you feel awful!

Some people say their affirmations out loud; others whisper them or sing them to themselves; still others just think them or find a chance to write them down. Some people write down their affirmations and then read them when they feel the need.

The scientific value of affirmations has been supported by studies done both with animals and with athletes. In both cases, performance improves with praise, not with punishment. A constant round of "Good for you" seems to help a tennis game far more than "Next time, try putting your foot farther forward."

If this idea intrigues you, we suggest you give it a try, just for a week. Find *something* to praise yourself for in everything you do, even if normally you'd feel critical. If you feel drawn to negative judgments, say to yourself, "That's for next week. This week is for my experiment." Then at the end of the week, see how you did. You may find that even your own high standards are easier to meet when you're affirming yourself!

Meditation

A variety of meditation techniques exist, including those associated with yoga and Zen Buddhism. Here, we describe the form known as transcendental meditation, or TM. TM involves focusing on a mantra, a single significant word. The focus allows your mind to free itself from its usual daily concerns. Ideally, your mantra is assigned by someone, but you may also use *om*, which means "whole," or, if you prefer English, *one*.

Find a comfortable place to sit. Straighten your spine, close your eyes, let your hands rest comfortably in your lap, and breathe deeply. Each time you exhale, repeat your mantra, either silently or aloud. If other thoughts intrude, allow them simply to pass through your mind.

Eventually, you can work up to ten to twenty minutes of meditation per day, once or twice a day. Many people find that besides offering relief from headache, meditation helps them center on their true concerns, feel more self-confident, and experience more joy.

BIOFEEDBACK

The forms of relaxation described so far all depend only on your own experience of your body. Biofeedback adds to that awareness an objective measurement, in which a machine measures the extent to which your scalp muscles are contracted, determines the circulation in your hands, or monitors the amount of blood pulsing through your temporal artery (the artery running through your temples) or through the arteries in your hand. As we indicate in Chapter 2, any of these locations might be involved in the chain of events that produces either a migraine or a tension-type headache. By receiving *feedback* about these *bio*logical processes, you can learn to modify them, thus affecting your headaches.

Biofeedback's Effectiveness

Biofeedback has been found to be extremely effective with migraine patients and with patients suffering from tension-type headache (apparently, it has been rather less effective in treating cluster headache). In one study, biofeedback relieved 70 percent of the chronic tension-type headaches in those who tried it (admittedly a highly motivated, self-selected group). Other studies found that it offered relief to as many as 60 percent of the migraineurs who tried it.

Biofeedback seems to be helpful both in preventing headaches and in responding to them once they have begun. When biofeedback is combined with relaxation techniques, it is even more effective. And its results seem to last. Follow-up studies of migraineurs have shown that a 57 to 70 percent improvement was maintained months or years after the first treatment.

One study of migraineurs divided subjects into four groups: those who received training in biofeedback plus relaxation techniques, those who received only biofeedback, those taught only relaxation techniques, and those who received a placebo — ineffective pills plus inaccurate information about their biofeedback experience. Some 65 percent of the group that was trained in both experienced some headache relief compared with 52 percent trained in biofeedback alone and 53 percent trained in relaxation techniques alone. (By the way, 17 percent experienced relief from the placebo, proving once again that the mind is a powerful healer!)

Of the patients suffering from tension-type headache, 61 percent of those who learned only biofeedback got some relief, as opposed to 59 percent of those who learned both techniques, 59 percent of those using only relaxation techniques, and 35 percent of those using the placebo.

The variation among the top three categories was very small in this single study, so these figures should not be used to evaluate the relative merits of biofeedback versus relaxation techniques. Rather, the figures show that both approaches are helpful. In our opinion, if these approaches are combined with changes in diet and patterns of regular aerobic exercise, the benefits become even greater.

How Biofeedback Works

Biofeedback is taught by a trained therapist, who generally begins treatment by giving you a detailed questionnaire about your headaches and your general health, as well as about your lifestyle, your diet, and the major areas of stress in your work and home life. (For more about the kind of information you should bring to any initial headache consultation, see Chapter 3.) You will probably be asked to keep a pain diary for four weeks or so, much like the headache calendar we ourselves recommend.

A therapist most likely will caution you not to expect the "fast, fast, fast relief" that television commercials promise for their medications. Rather, you are entering into a process that relies upon your awareness of your own body. As this awareness grows, so does your relief, but it's not something that can be learned in a day. On the other hand, the wide-ranging benefits of biofeedback can last you a lifetime!

The therapist will show you some biofeedback equipment that measures your muscle tone, blood flow, or hand temperature. You receive some type of feedback in the form of a beep, a meter, flashing lights, an oscillating tone, a digital readout, or perhaps the therapist's own reaction as he or she reads the machine. Thus, whenever you relax your muscles or raise the temperature of your hand (thus drawing more blood into it, away from your head), the tone lowers or the lights stop flashing.

Once you understand the feedback concept, your next step is to become aware of the relaxation state that the equipment has identified. Your goal is to feel what it's like to be truly relaxed. The theory is that once you can feel this state, you can duplicate it whenever you like, thus preventing or interrupting headaches.

A biofeedback therapist works with you in a variety of ways, perhaps teaching you some of the relaxation techniques described in this chapter: breathing exercises, progressive relaxation, guided imagery exercises, and autogenic suggestions. You will also be encouraged to develop a greater body awareness, so that you can identify when key muscles in your back, shoulder, neck, scalp, and face are tense and so that you can feel when your blood vessels are constricting. Over time, you and your therapist will discuss ways that you can heighten your own bodily awareness, perhaps keeping a debriefing log to record your experience with biofeedback or perhaps continuing to keep a headache calendar.

Some therapists provide patients with home biofeedback monitors, generally thermal rings that measure the heat in a finger. Again, if your hands are hot, chances are your head is not throbbing with excess blood painfully dilating blood vessels in and around the scalp.

Your therapist may also assign you mini-exercises, such as "Clench your jaw; now relax your jaw," "Tighten and relax your shoulders," or "Close your eyes for three minutes and imagine yourself on a warm, tropical beach. Feel the sun and hear the waves pounding on the beach." Many people find it helpful to check in with themselves in this way, stopping throughout the day to monitor where their bodies are tense and then working on those spots.

In some cases, you may return to your therapist for "booster" sessions some weeks or months after training has been completed. Clearly, biofeedback trains you in an active, lifelong process of relaxation and body awareness.

Biofeedback and Medication

Although the goal of biofeedback is to develop drug-free ways of preventing and treating headache, many people wonder whether they might try biofeedback without giving up their medication. The answer is yes, depending on the type of medication.

A person who is taking an occasional pain reliever, whether prescription or over-the-counter, can certainly benefit from biofeedback. However, if you are taking pain relievers of any kind more than three times per week, you may be suffering from the analgesic rebound effect, in which you become so dependent upon the pain reliever that you develop a headache as soon as the medication wears off. These frequent, even daily, headaches can be treated only by coming off the pain relievers: Biofeedback has little chance of success until the withdrawal process is complete. (For more information on the analgesic rebound effect, see Chapter 9.)

Likewise, benzodiazepines (tranquilizers such as Valium, Ativan, and Xanax) are at cross-purposes with biofeedback. Their effect is often to dull your awareness of your body, whereas biofeedback seeks to heighten awareness. For biofeedback to be effective, you need all of your faculties and responses intact.

Other types of medication, such as beta-blockers (e.g., propranolol HCl, or Inderal) and antidepressants (e.g., amitriptyline HCl, or Elavil), do not interfere with biofeedback, although beta-blockers may affect people's ability to learn how to warm their hands. Beta-blockers' side effects may include depression, so people who are thus affected may not benefit from biofeedback's tendency to make people feel empowered and in control of their lives.

The Side Effects of Biofeedback

People who practice biofeedback report improved sleep patterns, better moods, and a sense of empowerment and control. Ironically, while the side effects of drugs often include such side effects as depression and despondency, the side effects of biofeedback are all exclusively positive.

OTHER DRUG-FREE WAYS TO RELIEVE A HEADACHE

So far, we've focused on ways to enlist your mind in the effort to rid yourself of headaches. For the moment, let's get physical; that is, let's focus on purely physical, drug-free techniques that you can use when you feel a headache coming on. You can also use these techniques in conjunction with the other methods we've suggested.

Apply Heat or Cold

The general rule is that heat is good to apply *before* a headache. For migraineurs heat helps constricted blood vessels relax, while for tension-type headache sufferers it helps loosen the muscles.

Cold, on the other hand, is supposed to be better *during* a headache: It helps constrict the dilated blood vessels of a migraine attack and helps block the pain messages traveling to your brain. Since cold and pain travel along the same neural pathways to the brain, cold overrides the pain messages and thus brings some relief, numbing the area of application.

In addition, cold slows down biological processes. If your pain is heightened by the metabolic waste products left in your muscles (see Chapter 2), cold may slow down the production of this waste, thereby relieving some pain. Cold also decreases the incidence of muscle spasms that may cause pain.

However, ultimately, your own instincts are most reliable. Whichever method sounds more appealing to you is the one you should try first. You may need to use both.

Applying Heat

Find a way to sit or lie down that doesn't put any strain on your neck: lying on your back with a pillow below your knees and with a rolled-up towel below your neck, or sitting with your arms crossed on top of a table and with your forehead resting on your arms. Your goal in either case is total relaxation, allowing all your body to sink into the chair or the floor.

You might use a low-intensity moist heating pad, a very warm moist towel, or a hot-water bottle for no more than twenty minutes to an hour. (Longer might damage your skin.) Mentholated lotions may bring relief during your rest periods, which should last at least forty minutes.

You might also sit in the shower with your head resting on your arms, allowing hot water to beat on your head, shoulders, and neck. A towel draped over your shoulders may help the heat reach your body more evenly. Likewise, you could sit in a hot tub, resting your neck against a bath pillow, hot towel, or cushion. Don't throw your head back too far, or you will simply strain your neck in the other direction. If the skin on the back of your neck is wrinkled, it's bent too far.

You may wish to make hot compresses out of folded cotton towels, soaked in water as hot as you can stand it and then wrung out. Ideally, another person would apply these compresses, but you may apply your own if need be. Lie on your back in the position described above and apply one compress behind your neck, one across your forehead, and two over your collarbone, covering your shoulders. The towels should stay hot for about five minutes; reheat them and apply again, up to a total of twenty minutes of treatment. End with ten minutes of a hot compress covering your face, leaving only your nostrils free to breathe. Some people combine this treatment with one of the relaxation or visualization exercises described above. In any case, breathe deeply and slowly.

Applying Cold

If you like to feel prepared, leave a Styrofoam or paper cup full of water in the freezer, so that you can tear away the cup's top inch when you need a cold compress. If you prefer a more refined compress, buy a gel cold pack or cervical ice pillow at the drugstore and leave it in the freezer. For making compresses on the spot, you can wrap some ice cubes in a plastic bag and then in a damp towel, or you can leave a damp washcloth in the freezer for ten minutes or so.

Apply the cold to any place where you feel pain. Here are a few suggestions: your neck, the top of your head, the nape of your neck, and just below your occipital bone (the bone that sticks out in a bump on the back of your head [where your spine meets the back of your head]). Many important pain nerves from your brain and your spinal cord meet at an area two inches below the base of your skull, so you might apply cold to your upper cervical spine, numbing the area and slowing nerve transmission.

You might ask your doctor about obtaining a suboccipital ice pillow, a collarlike device with a thin slit in back in which you place a frozen gel pack. You then fit the collar around your neck, and ice the back of the skull and the upper neck. This device seems to be as effective as some medication in stopping a mild to moderate headache, as long as you use it early enough.

Acupressure

This self-help technique is a variation on the ancient Chinese practice of acupuncture, which corrects an imbalance of the two parts of a life force known as *ch'i*. In acupuncture, a trained practitioner inserts wire-thin needles at specific body points. Many people go to trained acupuncturists for treatment of headache and report good results for preventing headaches, improving sleep patterns, alleviating some aspects of depression, and creating a general feeling of well-being.

Although it takes years to learn acupuncture, you can learn some acupressure techniques in a few minutes. They're useful both when you feel a headache coming on and when you're in the midst of pain. You can also easily teach someone else to administer acupressure to you. It's all a matter of knowing where the pressure points are and administering three full minutes of firm pressure. It's important to give yourself the full three minutes, because you may not feel anything at all for most of that time — and then suddenly you may notice relief. However, if the pressure is causing pain, stop at once. Don't ever apply pressure to a swollen or infected area.

Next time you're feeling headachy, try applying pressure at these points: just above the top of the ear, in line with the ear canal; over the bony knobs in the back of the lower part of your skull; just in front of the place where the front of the upper part of your ear attaches to the scalp. Your head and your hands also correspond; that is, they share certain nerve centers, so you might try pressing the small muscle in the web space between your thumb and index finger (when you bring your thumb toward your index finger, that muscle stands out on the back side of your hand); or the web space between your little finger and ring finger.

Massage

Massage is helpful for both preventing and treating headaches. Although it's ideal to receive a massage from someone else, you can administer some kinds of self-massage also. To find a professional masseur, you might check out health food stores, dance studios, or newspaper advertisements. Possibly you can also get a reference from a friend, physician, physical therapist, or chiropractor. There are many different types of massage, so you may need to experiment and explore a bit before you find the form of .nassage that works best for you.

Massage courses are available through many adult education centers and through the YMCA-type organizations. Your own masseur may also be able to teach you something about self-massage.

Meanwhile, some suggestions for self-massage to combat an incipient headache follow.

Let your head drop, so that your chin rests almost on your chest. Put your palms on the back of your head and press, very gently, to stretch out your neck. Don't press too hard or strain your muscles, however. The goal is to imagine your neck muscles as loose and soft; don't fight them, but stroke them into softness.

Run your thumbs and fingers down the back of your neck,

occasionally shaking your head gently. Use visualization to help yourself relax; you might think of your head as a balloon full of air, so light that it can easily move from one side to the other.

Work your hands over your temples and ears to loosen your face and scalp. Brace your thumbs against your scalp and rotate them in small circles, pressing firmly. Try pressing your palms and the heels of your hands flat against the sides of your head, pressing as hard as you can on the soft parts of your skull. Don't press in, though, pull up; visualize yourself lifting the headache right out of your head.

Continue to rotate among these various methods as your instincts dictate. Remember, your goal is to keep your neck loose, so whenever you need to, shake your head gently from side to side. As you like, you might work on your shoulders a bit, picturing them as soft and loose while you gently rub them. You may be tempted to fight your body, pummeling it into softness; however, this won't make you any more relaxed!

You may also notice that the relaxation process releases a final wave of pain before you reach relief. If the pain is sudden, sharp, or different in any way from your former headache pain, stop immediately. If it is only an intensification of your previous headache, however, breathe deeply and continue. Our patients have often told us that their headaches peak most intensely just before finally passing.

Stretching

As with so many of the drug-free approaches to headache relief outlined here, stretching has benefits that go far beyond the treatment of headache. Stretching helps you stay flexible, a state that slows down the aging process. It helps your muscles relax and stimulates your circulation, both of which can help prevent headache and keep you in top physical condition.

Perhaps more importantly, taking a "stretch break" from your activities at work or at home can be your way of caring for yourself and focusing on your own needs, rather than being swept away by the needs and demands of others. If you think taking a few minutes to stretch every hour or two is just too much time away from your desk or apart from your kids, ask yourself what kind of statement you're making about your life and your own needs.

You can learn a variety of stretching routines from classes in yoga, t'ai chi, dance, or general exercise. We also provide one routine here. Start by keeping two things in mind:

- The goal is to lengthen and loosen your muscles, not to force your body into positions that are unnatural or uncomfortable.

- Keep breathing! It may be tempting to hold your breath while stretching, but don't. Explore the ways that inhaling and exhaling can help you extend or release your stretch.

Here's a routine that takes from ten to fifteen minutes. We suggest moving slowly and thoroughly, even if it means doing a bit less. You can certainly break up the routine into segments, doing, say, five minutes at a time over the course of your day. You can also focus on stretching the muscles that seem to be more tense at that time.

Begin in a standing position, barefoot or wearing flat shoes, feet apart, about the distance between your shoulders. Let your chin drop onto your chest. Then, gently, let your head fall back as your mouth opens. Not too far back — you don't want to strain your neck — just far enough to keep from wrinkling the skin on the back of your neck. Roll your head gently to the right, trying to touch right ear to right shoulder. Then roll front, then left, then repeat toward the right again. Then roll slowly and continuously in one direction for three to five rolls, repeating in the opposite direction for the same number of rolls. This is known as a neck roll.

After your neck roll, let your head float up into a centered, upright position. Stretch your shoulders by raising them, reaching for your ears. Let them drop and relax completely. Inhale on the rise and exhale on the drop. Remember, your goal is to stretch and relax, not to throw or force your muscles into a strained position. Repeat the shoulder stretch five or six times.

Now pull your shoulders forward, and then back, again moving gently but thoroughly. Repeat five or six times. Stay aware of your body, feeling the difference between moving your shoulders *forward* and moving them *up*.

Finally, rotate your shoulders so that one thrusts forward while the other thrusts back. Again, feel the difference between moving your shoulders and moving your arms; see how fully you can isolate your shoulders while keeping your arms and back relaxed. Visualize each part of your body floating into place, moving effortlessly. And keep breathing slowly and deeply!

Aerobic Exercise

Perhaps the single best way you can combat headache is to get twenty to thirty minutes of vigorous aerobic exercise four to five times a week. Aerobic exercise helps dispel stress, improve circulation, and move more oxygen to the brain. It also produces endorphins, which combat pain, create a sense of well-being, and treat depression. We have patients who have virtually eliminated frequent headaches, just by doing aerobic exercise five times a week.

Recommended exercise includes walking, running, bicycling, swimming, an aerobic sport such as singles tennis or racquetball, or an aerobics class. Several home machines can also be used, such as a stationary bike, treadmill, cross-country ski machine, stepper, and rowing machine. Your state of health may affect the form of exercise you choose, but most people can walk at a brisk pace for fifteen to twenty minutes at a time, five times a week. (If you are at all concerned about your ability to exercise, of course, check with your doctor.)

Weight lifting and other muscle-toning activities may have other health benefits, but they are not nearly as effective in preventing headache. Weight lifting tends to contract the muscles, and too-vigorous weight lifting may even cause headaches in some people. Nor is weight lifting aerobic exercise.

Generally, it's better to exercise moderately four or five times a week than to knock yourself out once or twice a week. The goal is to raise the entire level of your body's functioning, which is best done by regular activity.

Studies have shown that moderate aerobic exercise for twenty to thirty minutes, three times a week, prolongs life and decreases the likelihood of some types of cancer and heart problems. However, the benefits don't seem to go up with more exercise; really, a moderate amount of exercise regularly is all you need. We suggest exercising more often mainly as a way of dissipating the stress that can often trigger a headache. It also brings you personal time and respite from the more hectic activities of daily life.

HEADACHE AND EMOTIONAL ISSUES

For most of this chapter, we've dealt with various techniques for coping with stress. Now let's look at some of the sources of stress in women's lives and at some of the ways that women may use headaches to "speak" for them.

Two renowned headache researchers have postulated about psychological aspects of migraine. Harold Wolff, a rather authoritative personality, spoke of migraine as a "biologic reprimand" for overdoing it; John Graham, a rather gentle person, referred to migraine as "angina of the soul." Although we certainly don't believe that anyone would consciously induce the pain of a headache, psychoanalysts may think that a woman might come to believe, perhaps without realizing it, that she can communicate needs through her headache that she can't express in any other way. In psychological language, these needs are known as *secondary gains,* the gains that someone gets "in exchange" for a painful problem. Although the secondary gains may not be the source of the problem — as we've discussed, a biochemical predisposition might be the ultimate source of headache — secondary gains may help to keep a problem in place.

For example, let's imagine that a married woman with three children works as an office manager. Her sense of herself as a wife, mother, and friend demands that she put others' needs before her own. At work she's aware that many of the male executives above her don't take her very seriously, while many of the female secretaries below her resent her, both as a boss and as a woman who has risen above them.

Let's further suppose that this woman was born with a biological predisposition to migraine. She starts with a physiological tendency to translate any stresses that come up at home or at work into headaches, unless she consciously commits to overcoming this tendency through careful management of diet, regular exercise, and attention to relaxation techniques. Even in the absence of particular psychological issues, she finds this commitment difficult: her husband and kids are always wanting something when she's at home, her job is quite demanding, and she can't quite see finding private downtime away from the people she works with or lives with to give herself regular ten-minute "relaxation" breaks. It just isn't going to happen.

So what happens instead? Periodically, she gets headaches so intense that she is confined to bed. Although she dearly loves her children, she can't see them while her head hurts, and her husband has to either make sure he's home to take care of them or arrange for alternative child care. Although she loves her husband, too, it's clear that she just can't think about him while she's in bed with a migraine, although both of them know she'll make it up to him afterward. Although she's dedicated to her job, she doesn't believe she can control the fact that sometimes she just gets sick.

One way to look at this woman's headaches, then, is to see them as her only language for saying no. Since she can't, in her perception, take relaxation breaks at work or carve out more time for herself at home, her body finds another way of getting moments of rest and privacy. Of course, "time out" with a throbbing migraine isn't exactly a vacation or a happy day off, but on some level, terrible pain may be the only way for this woman to get rest and privacy and maybe even sympathy and attention. These benefits are called *secondary* gains — because they result from the primary condition, a headache.

Following this reasoning, if the woman could learn to listen to her body more carefully, she might be able to say no more often and earlier. Then she wouldn't have to say no with her body, through a headache, to get what she needs.

It may be that everyone sees this woman as a tower of strength — she may even see herself that way — so the only time her vulnerability, her weaknesses, and her needs are acknowledged is when she gets sick. These are her secondary gains.

However, if she could find ways of saying in words or in other actions, "Sometimes I get scared; sometimes I feel overwhelmed; sometimes I need to be taken care of," she might find herself taking other actions that would keep her from getting so many headaches. She might make time to talk about her feelings with her husband, a friend, or a counselor. She might discover allies at work who could support her in her difficult position. She might decide that her current job is not for her and choose a kind of work where she's less isolated. As long as her headaches are "speaking for her," however, she's less likely to take action. She'll let the headaches do the talking — and she'll pay the terrible price of pain.

Our point is not that the woman is "bringing her headaches on herself," rather that there might be actions she could take to prevent the headaches, actions that she's not yet willing to take. If she could find other ways of getting more of what she wants, she might start a process that would lead to, among other things, having fewer headaches. Partly this result would be because she would no longer need her headaches to speak for her; she'd be speaking for herself.

What other ways might women use headache to speak for them? Below are some that we've observed.

Headaches as Anger

There are two ways of looking at "anger headaches," both of which may be true. One is to see anger as a source of stress that, like all sources of stress, is a potential headache trigger. The other is to see the headache itself as an angry act, a way of acting out hostility and despair when a woman doesn't think she has any other way to express her feelings.

Women in our society are frequently enjoined not to feel angry and certainly not to show their anger. "Bitch," "ball-buster," "harpy," "harridan," and "shrew" are just some of the words for an angry woman. Significantly, there are virtually no equivalent terms for an angry man.

Consequently, women with migraine may feel extra layers of stress around their anger. First, the anger itself is a stressor. Then the effort to suppress it may cause stress. Finally, the guilt at feeling angry — and the anger at having to suppress it! — add further levels of tension and strain.

If you think your headaches may be related to anger in some way, we suggest that you complete the following sentences. You can do it now, in your mind, as you're reading, or you might write out your answers in a diary or journal.

Self-Check on Anger

When I get angry, I express it by _____.
Right now, the person I'm most angry at is _____
   because _____.
I'm most often angry at _____ because
_____.
When my spouse/mate makes me angry, I respond by
_____. When I think of my re-
   sponse, I feel _____.
When my friend makes me angry, I respond by
_____. When I think of my re-
   sponse, I feel _____.
When my kids make me angry, I respond by
_____. When I think of my re-
   sponse, I feel _____.
When my boss makes me angry, I respond by
_____. When I think of my re-
   sponse, I feel _____.
When my coworker makes me angry, I respond by
_____. When I think of my re-
   sponse, I feel _____.
One way I would like to handle my anger differently is
_____.
I think angry people are _____.

Next, think of the last four or five times you were angry at someone. Write them in one column. Now think of the last four or five times you had a headache. Write the occasions in another column. Did any of the people you were angry with suffer in any way because of your headaches? Or did you yourself suffer as a result of getting angry? As you look at your lists, do you imagine that you got your headaches *instead* of getting angry, instead of either expressing your anger to the person involved or taking positive action to correct the situation?

Of course, it's not always possible or desirable to express your anger directly to the person involved, nor is action always a possibility. If you're in a lot of situations where your anger and your action are blocked, however, the stress may be triggering painful headaches. It might be worthwhile to give the matter some more thought, by writing in your journal, talking to a friend, or working with a counselor, to see if there are ways that you can act or express yourself more fully.

Headaches to Say No

As with our hypothetical woman, many women find it hard to say no. Some of this reluctance is internalized training; women are traditionally taught to value connections with others above their own sense of themselves, as well as being taught that "a real woman" nurtures and cares for others.

Sometimes, though, women find it hard to say no because they know they'll be punished for it, by parents, children, mates, friends, and, particularly, bosses and coworkers. Both women and men probably find it easier to hear no from a man than from a woman, and certainly at many work situations, women are expected to prove themselves by doing everything they are asked to do — and more!

In either case, a woman's frustration, exhaustion, and sense of being overwhelmed are all definitely stressors that could trigger a headache. Whether a woman doesn't want to fall short of her own "superwoman" standards or whether she feels others will punish her for setting limits, she still may feel obliged to do more than she wants to or is capable of doing, at work or at home.

Again, we might view the resulting headaches as triggered by the stress and the overwork. Or we might say that falling down sick with a headache is the only way a woman is "allowed"— whether by herself or others — to say no. Either way, if you think your headaches might be related to difficulties with saying no, take the following self-check, in your mind or in your journal:

Self-Check on Saying No

In my opinion, it's all right to say no if _____.
In my opinion, it's *not* all right to say no if _____.
The last three times I said no were 1. _____.
                                                 2. _____.
                                                 3. _____.
The last three times I *wanted* to say no were
                                                 1. _____.
                                               2. _____.
                                               3. _____.
The last three times I got a headache were
                                               1. _____.
                                               2. _____.
                                               3. _____.

Does taking this self-check give you any insight into reasons you might be getting headaches? Again, if you think you see room for exploration, you might want to look further at this issue, alone, with a friend, or with a therapist. Once you can find ways of saying no that work for you, you might be able to avoid a good many of the headaches you're getting now.

Headaches for Nurturance

Traditionally, women are expected by themselves and others to be the caretakers and the nurturers. Getting sick may be one of the only times that a grown woman has anybody else taking care of her.

As with our previous examples, it may be that the strain of always needing to be strong and nurturing takes its toll, and that toll triggers a headache. Or it may be that on some level, a woman might need so deeply to be nurtured that she's willing to pay the price of a terrible headache if she believes it's the only way she can get what she wants. If a woman feels guilty about wanting to be cared for, she might think that the headache is an appropriate price to pay. If she fears punishment for having needs, she might think that having a headache may placate anyone who might be mad at her.

If you think your headaches might have something to do with needing nurturance, try taking the following self-check:

Self-Check on Nurturance

When someone else takes care of me, I feel _____.

The person who most often takes care of me when I get sick or need help is _____.

When I think of how that person feels about taking care of me, I imagine he or she feels _____.

When I think of what that person thinks of me, I imagine him or her as thinking _____.

How *I* feel about that person taking care of me is _____.

The feeling of being cared for is _____.

You might also list the last three or four times you felt fragile or overwhelmed, and then the last three or four times you got a headache. Do you notice any connection?

Getting the Help You Deserve

Once again, we strongly urge you to get help dealing with these issues if they seem important to you. Psychotherapists, religious counselors, family therapists, couples counselors, and therapy groups may all offer ways of exploring these and other concerns. There *are* ways of getting what you need, caring for yourself, and avoiding many of your headaches. It may take some time and commitment to figure out how, but you can do it — and you *deserve* to do it.

CHAPTER 9

Medicating Migraines

E VEN IF YOUR HEADACHES RESPOND TO DIET,
exercise, and behavioral approaches, you may often find
that you need medication to prevent or manage your
headaches. Such medication is, of course, available only by
doctor's prescription. You should also discuss with your
doctor any nonprescription medications you are taking. However, you are better able to take an active role in your own
treatment if you know about the medications now commonly
used to prevent and treat headache. This chapter offers you a
general overview of the latest pharmacological treatments
available to treat headache symptoms, abort a headache, or
prevent one altogether.

WHAT DOES MEDICATION DO?

Headache medication can interact with your body in four
basic ways:

- It may affect the biochemistry of your brain, increasing
  the availability of certain neurotransmitters and
  counteracting the biochemical chain of events that leads
  to a headache.

- It may affect your blood vessels, encouraging them either
  to constrict or to dilate, or reducing inflammation around
  them.

- It may modify muscle tone, causing tight muscles to relax or preventing muscles from contracting in the first place.

- It may elevate your pain threshold — that is, the physical operation of the headache remains the same, but your experience of the pain is blocked or diminished.

At times, these objectives may be achieved by the nondrug methods described in the previous two chapters. On the other hand, medication is often the fastest way to remove either pain or the threat of pain from a person's life. And sometimes that form of relief is needed to make room for other types of approaches.

We're aware that medications may have side effects. We also believe that a strong doctor-patient partnership, in which patients are actively reporting to doctors and doctors are viewing patients as whole people (rather than as sets of symptoms), can negotiate those dangers and provide patients with safe, effective headache relief through medication.

To that end, we offer the following overview. Knowing what types of medication are available and learning something about the pros and cons of each helps make you a more active — and effective — partner in your own treatment.

GENERAL PRINCIPLES OF PHARMACOLOGIC TREATMENT

You have to be careful not to overuse symptomatic or abortive headache medications (the different types of headache medication are described in detail below). Using analgesics, ergotamine tartrate, barbiturates, or sedatives on a consistent basis can lead to a *rebound syndrome*. At The New England Center for Headache we spend a lot of time taking patients off medication because they are already rebounding when they come to see us. So they will not overuse medications, we ask patients to keep a calendar of their headaches and the medications they are taking. A physician discusses the calendar with the patient on each revisit.

Rebound Headaches

It has been shown that taking two to four aspirin or acetaminophen tablets per day can lead to analgesic rebound headache. Stronger medications containing barbiturates or opiates (narcotics) and ergotamine tartrate are even worse offenders. The frequency with which one takes these medications each week is more important than the total dose per day. Therefore, we suggest that patients take pain medications no more than three days a week and use ergotamine tartrate no more than one or two days per week. Following these simple rules keeps a patient from developing a rebound syndrome with the resultant worsening of her headaches.

Patients who develop analgesic rebound headache have more severe and more perpetual headache and find that preventive medications and behavioral treatments are not helpful. The analgesic rebound effect is explained in greater detail below.

Side Effects

It is essential that patients understand why they are taking a medication, how to take it, and what the possible side effects might be. All medications have possible side effects, and headache medications often have strong side effects. We like to discuss the most common ones with patients and to hand them a sheet listing other possible side effects. We also tell them when to be concerned, when to call for help, when to go to the emergency room, and what to ask for when they arrive.

To avoid the side effects of preventive medication, we usually start with one medication at a time — in the lowest dose available and raise the dose slowly over a period of several weeks.

Timing

Every body is unique, and every nervous system reacts differently to medication. Some patients find that a particular medicine taken before bedtime makes them hyper, prevents them from sleeping, and is ineffective. Another person taking the same dose of the same medication may find that it puts her to sleep, makes her feel well rested in the morning, and takes away her headache. We tell patients what we expect of a medication but warn them that we cannot always predict accurately their reaction to a given medication.

In addition, we let our patients understand that there is always a period of adjustment for a daily medication. During the first two weeks the dose is usually too low to work, and the medication has not been given long enough to work. During the first few days of a new medication, there may be side effects that the body will adapt to. We therefore urge patients to stick to treatments unless the side effects are severe.

SYMPTOMATIC, ABORTIVE, AND PREVENTIVE MEDICATION

Medication can address your headache pain in one of three ways:

- It can address the *symptoms* of your pain, rather than the underlying mechanisms that caused the pain in the first place. Most off-the-shelf medication is *symptomatic* medication of this type.

- It can *abort* a headache that has already begun or is just about to begin, by interfering with the underlying mechanisms that cause headache. *Abortive* medications generally must be prescribed by a physician.

- It can *prevent* a headache from beginning in the first place — or, more conservatively, can reduce the frequency, duration, and severity of headache attacks. *Preventive* medication must always be prescribed by a physician. Sometimes your doctor will prescribe only one type, sometimes more than one. You need to know what he or she is prescribing and why. There are nonprescription agents available that may help prevent a headache like feverfew, magnesium, vitamins B_2 and B_6, and spirulina (which contains 500 mg tryptophan).

Symptomatic Medication

If you take off-the-shelf medication regularly, you have in effect been prescribing symptomatic medication for yourself. A physician may also have been treating your headaches with high doses of ibuprofen or some combination of *analgesic* plus *narcotic* (now termed "opiate") — for example, Tylenol with codeine, Fiorinal with codeine. Some *analgesics* relieve pain without affecting consciousness; while others, such as opiates, relieve pain and may dull consciousness, producing drowsiness.

You may be responding well to the occasional use of symptomatic medication, whether prescribed or off-the-shelf. In our experience, however, because this type of medication doesn't really address the underlying cause of headaches, it tends to lose its effectiveness when taken too regularly or in too large a quantity. Consequently, many patients tend to overuse it, with the result that their headaches may actually increase in severity and/or frequency. A very select group of refractory patients, however, may require ongoing opiate therapy. (For more on this syndrome, see the section on the analgesic rebound effect below.)

Abortive Medication

Severe headaches may require abortive medication. However, this type of medication may be associated with the greatest possibilities of overuse, and, ironically, the biggest chance of causing you *more* headache pain. As explained in more detail in the section on the analgesic rebound effect below, certain pain relievers may become necessary to your body, so that as the dosage wears off, your body develops a headache.

Abortive medication may be taken in tablet form. In some cases, though, tablets take too long to be fully absorbed by the stomach and small intestine — so that the medication never reaches the bloodstream. In migraine attacks, for example, changes in gastrointestinal activity may slow down the absorption of medication, even though the medication would have been effective could it have reached the blood. In those cases, abortive medication might have to be administered in the form of nasal sprays, suppositories, or injections preceded by medication that enhances absorption.

Most patients discover quickly that even medications effective in stopping a headache will not work if taken late in the course of the attack. We therefore suggest that medication be taken early in the attack, as soon as the headache begins to escalate in severity. This may also help to prevent overusing medication.

Preventive Medication

When headaches come more often than two or three times a month, when abortive medication doesn't seem to work, or when abortive medication is contraindicated because of another physical condition, preventive medication may be prescribed. These medications are not painkillers and usually take several weeks to build up in the nervous system before becoming effective. Therefore, we instruct our patients not to become frustrated by a medication's seeming ineffectiveness in the first two to three weeks, when the dose is being raised slowly. We and our patients have had remarkable success in relieving headache pain with preventive medication, a success that is supported by the findings of other doctors and researchers.

OFF-THE-SHELF VS. PRESCRIPTION DRUGS

Many people have the mistaken impression that if you can buy a drug without a doctor's prescription, its side effects are minimal or negligible. They also make the mistake of thinking that doctors aren't interested in a patient's use of nonprescription drugs.

In fact, many powerful headache remedies are available without a doctor's prescription, medications that can drastically affect your headache patterns, your general state of health, and your response to the medication that a doctor prescribes. If a doctor is prescribing preventive headache medication, for example, its effects may actually be sabotaged if you take a few aspirin or something stronger every time you feel the beginnings of a headache.

It's absolutely essential that you share full, detailed information with your doctor about your use of off-the-shelf medication. If you take a pain reliever stronger than aspirin or if you take aspirin more than twice a week, we strongly suggest that you keep a written record of your use of medication for two to three weeks before your next doctor's appointment and that you share this information with your physician. You may not realize how often you've been turning to Tylenol, Aleve, Advil, or Excedrin, nor how many tablets you usually take on a headachy day.

On the other hand, it's equally essential for your doctor to share with you the full story of any medication that he or she prescribes for you. Every individual's biochemistry is unique, and what affects your spouse or your neighbor one way may affect you in quite another. If your doctor is not letting you know what to expect from the medication you're being given, or if he or she doesn't seem interested in descriptions of your physical and emotional responses to it, you might bring up the matter. If things don't improve, you may need to find a more receptive doctor.

TYPES OF NONPRESCRIPTION MEDICATION

As we have seen, nonprescription medication is *symptomatic:* It acts to relieve only the symptoms of headache and in no way affects the underlying processes that cause headache.

Aspirin

Although aspirin is one of the most oft-taken pain relievers in the United States, nobody really knows exactly how it works. Aspirin prevents blood platelets from clumping together, which appears to be part of the migraine process.

Perhaps more importantly, aspirin seems to block the body's ability to synthesize prostaglandins. As we explain in Chapter 2, prostaglandins dilate blood vessels and produce pain and inflammation. So aspirin may interrupt headache by keeping prostaglandins from dilating blood vessels; aspirin may also raise our pain threshold by preventing prostaglandins from being manufactured. Recent research shows that aspirin may have an effect on serotonin.

Many off-the-shelf alternatives to aspirin are really only aspirin (acetylsalicylic acid) in another form. Anacin, for example, is aspirin plus 32 mg of caffeine. (For more on how caffeine may combat headache — or worsen it when overused — see Chapter 7.) And "extra strength" aspirin is only aspirin in a larger dose. Consumers do tend to up their dosage from one to two or even three tablets, however, no matter what the actual strength of each tablet may be.

Aspirin's Side Effects Sometimes aspirin irritates the mucous membrane that lines the digestive tract. People who take aspirin daily (*not* recommended for chronic headache patients in any case!) experience some distress 2 to 10 percent of the time. People who take ten tablets a day or more experience marked gastric distress 30 to 50 percent of the time. However, no headache patient should be taking that much aspirin in the first place. (See the section on analgesic rebound effect below.)

Aspirin is an anticoagulant and can have antiplatelet effects: It helps prevent the blood from clotting properly and thus can produce prolonged bleeding. These effects are why people with ulcers are warned off aspirin. In some cases, this anticoagulant effect can be relatively minor — patients may notice that they bruise easily — in other cases, it can cause a life-threatening condition, such as a bleeding ulcer.

People who take moderate to high doses of aspirin sometimes have *occult* (invisible) blood in their stools. For menstruating women, who are already losing blood, the anticoagulant effect may aggravate a tendency to anemia. In any case, two-thirds of those who *overuse* aspirin on a regular basis experience some degree of blood loss.

Some people have strong gastrointestinal reactions to aspirin. People who are sensitive to aspirin may also be sensitive to foods that contain *salicin*, one of its components. Such foods include apples, oranges, and bananas. People who are sensitive to aspirin may also react strongly to certain processed foods, as well as to some medications containing tartrazine dye, sodium benzoate, and iodide-containing agents. Peptic ulcers may be aggravated by these reactions.

Aspirin tends to concentrate in the kidneys, where it can cause kidney damage if the cumulative doses have been high enough.

Some people have a type of asthma that makes them aspirin-sensitive; some people even without asthma may react to aspirin with gasping, wheezing, or shortness of breath. In some cases, high dose of aspirin damages the eighth nerve, the hearing nerve, so that people suffer tinnitus, or ringing in the ears, as a result.

Tylenol: Effectiveness and Side Effects

Like aspirin, acetaminophen — known commercially as Tylenol — seems to affect our perception of pain. Unlike aspirin, however, it does *not* affect our blood-vessel activity and has only minimal anti-inflammatory effects. Tylenol's effects appear to be more central (brain).

Consumers often want to evaluate the relative merits of aspirin and Tylenol. To be honest, it's difficult to say. Aspirin's anti-inflammatory and antiplatelet effects may be more effective in combating migraine, especially when combined with caffeine. Like most consumers, you should probably just try different products until you find the one that works best for you.

Since different people respond differently to Tylenol, we can't tell you whether it or aspirin is more effective for *you*. However, we can share with you some information about Tylenol's side effects. Unfortunately, its side effects are not always visible, so you may be experiencing problems with Tylenol without being aware of them.

Too much Tylenol, especially when combined with alcohol, can cause liver damage. A sudden massive overdose of Tylenol can be reversed if the person takes an antidote — Mucomyst (acetylcysteine) — within eight to twenty-four hours. Pediatricians have come to rely on Tylenol because in children with fever, aspirin is associated with Reye's syndrome (a liver dysfunction in children who take aspirin), whereas Tylenol poses no such risk.

Tylenol has been available to adults only since 1974, when it was first marketed as a prescription drug. Chronic usage of Tylenol may also strain the liver, albeit in a way that takes some time to come to light. People who consume alcohol regularly should be cautious with Tylenol, or any medication. Tylenol is safer than aspirin in patients with asthma, bleeding disorders, ulcers, or heartburn and in pregnancy.

Ibuprofen: Effectiveness and Side Effects

Marketed as Advil, Motrin, or Nuprin, ibuprofen is classed with aspirin as a nonsteroidal anti-inflammatory drug (NSAID), that is, as a drug that raises our pain threshold and may in some way keep blood vessels from dilating. Also like aspirin, ibuprofen seems to inhibit our body's synthesis of prostaglandins. Since prostaglandins cause pain and inflammation while causing our blood vessels to dilate, it seems that inhibiting their synthesis would help interrupt headache pain.

Ibuprofen first came on the market in 1974 as Motrin, a prescription medication, and began to be marketed aggressively as an off-the-shelf medication under other names in 1983, such as Advil and Nuprin. Since ibuprofen works so much like aspirin, it's probably safe to assume that a sensitivity to one may indicate a sensitivity to the other. However, we know only a few specific side effects. For example, although ibuprofen may seem to cause less gastrointestinal distress than aspirin, overuse may lead to gastrointestinal discomfort, bleeding, or perforation.

Higher doses of ibuprofen are available by prescription only. If you are taking more than four to six tablets in twenty-four hours, or if you are taking any amount of ibuprofen more than three days per week, you may be "overprescribing" yourself. Besides putting yourself at risk for the analgesic rebound effect (see below), you may be at risk for gastrointestinal side effects. Rather than taking ibuprofen on a regular basis, you would probably benefit more by looking into other ways to prevent your headaches. There is controversy as to whether NSAIDs (other than aspirin) can cause rebound headaches.

Sinus Headache Remedies

As noted in Chapter 2, few headaches are likely to be caused by sinus problems, although you may feel pain in your sinuses. Sinus headache medications are usually some combination of caffeine, if used regularly, or decongestant plus an analgesic. We've already seen how caffeine may have headache-producing side effects. In addition, the decongestant may increase your blood pressure or otherwise affect your circulation, both problem areas for people with headache.

In our opinion, if you experience sinus pain along with headache pain and you're looking for an off-the-shelf remedy, you'd do better with plain aspirin, Tylenol, ibuprofen, or small amounts of sinus medication plus cutting down on dairy products. As we discuss in Chapter 7, dairy products, especially milk, cause you to produce phlegm and mucus, which can give you that "clogged-head" feeling, especially on damp, "headachy" days.

You should not be taking sinus medication more than three or four times a month, at most. If you feel the need for relief more often than that, discuss your condition with your doctor. In any case, if you are taking off-the-shelf sinus medication, the physician treating you for headache should be aware of it.

Combination Off-the Shelf Medications

Most combination off-the-shelf drugs basically contain an analgesic plus caffeine. Many studies indicate that caffeine is an adjuvant and may boost the pain-relieving effect when combined with aspirin and Tylenol or with aspirin alone. Excedrin, Cope, Midol, Vanquish, and Maximum Strength Anacin fit this formula.

Although caffeine can boost the pain-relieving properties of aspirin or aspirin combined with Tylenol (e.g., Excedrin), some people may be very sensitive to caffeine. For those people, caffeine *used in excess* can cause nausea, dizziness, anxiety, and sleeplessness. When the caffeine wears off, users can feel groggy, drowsy, lethargic, irritable, and depressed. They may also suffer from a caffeine-withdrawal headache!

Combine these side effects with those of analgesics, and you can see why you shouldn't be taking any off-the-shelf medication more than two or three times a week without discussing it with your doctor. And, of course, if your doctor is prescribing other headache medication, he or she needs to know if you *ever* take off-the-shelf medication.

Some headache preparations include an analgesic plus a mild sedative, for example, Excedrin PM, Tylenol PM, Cope, Midol, and Percogesic. The sedative does not affect the headache or the pain in any way; it only helps you sleep. If used too frequently, it may also create a rebound effect, so that you develop more headaches as soon as you stop taking the medication.

THE ANALGESIC REBOUND EFFECT

The notion of analgesic rebound effect is probably the single most important concept that anyone who takes off-the-shelf medication needs to understand. Far from simply relieving headaches, all pain relievers — analgesics — can also set you up to have *more* headaches.

How? It's simple. If your body comes to rely on analgesics, it actually develops headaches to signal its desire for more medication. Rather than taking pills to treat a headache, you find yourself taking them simply by *prevent* a headache from getting worse as the pain-medication levels decrease in your body. Taking more pills does not bring you more relief (except, perhaps, for a few hours). It will, however, "teach" your body to rely on analgesics.

Thus, many people with severe headache find themselves taking aspirin, Tylenol, ibuprofen, or Aleve several days per week, even daily. If you are taking any such medication more than three days a week, you are probably suffering from the analgesic rebound effect. As soon as the medication starts to wear off, you get another headache, signaling your body's desire for more. Iboprofen and Aleve may not contribute to rebound.

The analgesic rebound effect may occur with any other type of analgesic, whether off-the-shelf or prescription. Your clue is the amount of medication you are taking: If you take them more than three days per week, your pills may be causing more headaches than they relieve. If you suspect this analgesic rebound effect may be a problem for you, make sure to see a doctor who understands this condition. He or she can work with you to get you off the medication safely and comfortably (though you may have to tolerate some increased headache pain for a time), while helping you to find drug and nondrug relief that works better for you.

TYPES OF PRESCRIPTION MEDICATIONS

ABORTIVE MEDICATION FOR MIGRAINE

Abortive drugs are used to reduce the intensity and duration of headache pain, as well as to treat the associated symptoms of nausea, vomiting, and light sensitivity. Even more than symptomatic medications, some have a tendency to produce dependency and a rebound effect and may cause an increased frequency of headache. Furthermore, they may actually interfere with the effectiveness of preventive headache medication. Consequently, you should work closely with your physician to monitor your use of abortive medication and its effect on your health, lifestyle, and general sense of well-being.

Following are some commonly prescribed abortive medications.

Ergotamine tartrate

Ergotamine tartrate has been one of the most effective migraine-abortive drugs over the last fifty years. It causes the arteries to constrict, reduces inflammation, and stimulates serotonin receptors on nerves and blood vessels.

As we explain in Chapter 2, a migraine begins secondary to biochemical changes in the brain and in some cases is associated with an "aura" of visual or sensory disturbances. In addition, blood vessels dilate excessively, filling with too much blood, and contributing to the throbbing pain of the headache. (For more detail on this process, see Chapter 2.) Hence, medications that interrupt this process by causing the arteries to constrict are known as *vasoconstrictors*.

Vasoconstrictors must be taken at the first sign of a migraine, when the blood vessels are getting ready to dilate. They abort headaches by preventing dilation of blood vessels and stimulating serotonin receptors.

Ergotamines are available in various forms, most commonly, as *ergotamine tartrate* (Cafergot, Wigraine*)* and *dihydroergotamine (*D.H.E. 45*)*. Ergot compounds should be taken at the first sign of a migraine. About 90 percent of those patients who use ergotamines find that they work in twenty to sixty minutes. Some 80 percent of users find that rectal suppositories work the fastest; some 50 percent of users find that tablets do. Some patients prefer to inhale ergot compounds or to take them under the tongue.

Ergot compounds seem to act in three places:

- on the centers of the brain that regulate the arteries
- on the nerves that carry information about pain to the brain
- on the blood vessels themselves to constrict them and reduce inflammation

Therefore, people with high blood pressure should use this type of medication cautiously and not at all if blood pressure is uncontrolled. People suffering from certain heart or blood vessel diseases, people older than age fifty, or people with any type of brain disease, such as lupus, should also be cautious about using this medication.

Unfortunately, some ergotamines can produce or worsen nausea. Antiemetics (drugs that combat nausea and vomiting) can prevent the nausea produced by ergotamine. A drug like metoclopramide (Reglan), promethazine (Phenergan), or prochlorperazine (Compazine) should be taken fifty to thirty minutes before the ergotamine, if nausea is to be prevented.

Metoclopramide also helps empty the stomach and enhances the absorption of other medications administered with it. Promethazine doesn't help empty the stomach but does help control nausea and vomiting. Dimenhydrinate chloropmil (Dramamine), trimethobenzamide (Tigan), and hydroxyzine (Vistaril) are also effective antiemetics.

Bellergal is a combination of ergotamine tartrate, an antinausea drug, and a barbiturate sedative — a powerful but potentially problematic combination. We are extremely cautious about prescribing it. It can be used for a week at a time or to treat a menstrual headache, but as with other ergots its use should be limited to twice a week to prevent rebound headaches. Bellergal should not be used on an ongoing basis, except in certain circumstances.

In addition, 5 to 10 percent of those who use ergotamines experience the following side effects: abdominal or chest pain, muscle cramps, vertigo or dizziness, or coldness and tingling in the limbs. *Be sure to tell your doctor if you experience any such effects.*

People who take ergotamine compounds too frequently may accumulate high levels of ergots in their systems and develop *ergotism.* This rare syndrome may include cramps, chest pain, changes in the heart rate, numbness, tingling, pallor, decreased pulses, swelling in the extremities, epileptic seizures, changes in vision and temperature, mood disturbances, confusion, and hallucinations, all potentially caused by this vasoconstrictor's ability to reduce the flow of blood to the brain and the extremities or possibly by its effects on the brain's chemistry. Ergot comes from a rye fungus, and there's some evidence that those tried for witchcraft in seventeenth-century Salem were suffering from ergotism-related hallucinations.

Dihydroergotamine (D.H.E. 45)

Dihydroergotamine is a derivative of ergotamine that produces only modest arterial constriction. As a result, this type of drug has less of a detectable effect on the flow of blood to the brain. However, it may be even more effective than ergotamine tartrate for many. Some researchers have found that D.H.E. seems to act at sites in the brain stem (in the back of the brain) that are central to producing migraine as well as acting directly on blood vessels and nerve terminals.

Dihydroergotamine is currently available only as an injection, although a nasal spray preparation named Migranal is being evaluated by the FDA. Patients can be taught to self-inject D.H.E. under the skin, but most will prefer the nasal spray; it also is much less likely to produce rebound than ergotamine tartrate.

Some researchers have found success in combining D.H.E. with prochlorperazine (Compazine), administering 5 mg of prochlorperazine and 0.75 mg of D.H.E. intravenously over several minutes in the emergency room, perhaps giving another 0.5 mg of D.H.E. after sixty minutes. We ourselves have had success with 1 mg of D.H.E. plus 50 mg of promethazine (Phenergan), plus 4 mg of dexamethsone (Decadron) in intractable headache situations. These are given as three separate intramuscular shots. The D.H.E. can also be self-administered at home subcutaneously, or under the skin, as mentioned.

We consider D.H.E. one of the most effective migrainal treatments in an emergency-room setting or office, because it acts so quickly and with so few side effects.

Sumatriptan

Sumatriptan (Imitrex) is a major innovation in the acute treatment of migraine. It was released in early 1993 in the United States as a subcutaneous (under the skin) injection and is now available in tablet form. The 6 mg, self-injectable dose stops migraine in approximately thirty to sixty minutes in 70 to 80 percent of patients who try it. In a study done at The New England Center for Headache and published in the journal *Headache*, 84 percent of the patients studied had almost no headache within forty minutes. Eighty-one percent of the patients studied said it was the best medication they had taken for migraine. Many of them had minor side effects that lasted less than thirty minutes. The tablet takes somewhat longer to work and may work on slightly fewer patients.

The dose of the injectable medication is 6 mg, and another dose can be used within twenty-four hours if the headache either does not go away or goes away but recurs. Patients should not use more than two injections per day and four injections per week (but an absolute maximum of six injections per week is sometimes permitted). The tablet is available in 25 or 50 mg strengths. Twenty-five or 50 mg should be taken and may be repeated if the headache recurs, up to a total of 300 mg in twenty-four hours.

The side effects of the injection include pain at the injection site, tingling in the hands and feet, a warm or flushed feeling all over, an unusual feeling inside the body (as though something is traveling in the blood vessels), and a tightness or heaviness in the chest or throat. Side effects of the tablet are similar except for injection-site reactions. Because the drug is a strong constrictor of blood vessels, the first dose in patients over the age of forty should be taken in a physician's office. If patients develop tightness or heaviness in the chest, they should have a cardiogram to make sure they are not having constriction of the coronary arteries. The drug is contraindicated for patients with a history of heart disease, chest pain, uncontrolled high blood pressure, or stroke and for patients with several risk factors for cardiac disease (high cholesterol, lack of exercise, obesity, high blood pressure, and history of smoking). Patients should not take ergotamine tartrate or D.H.E. and sumatriptan in the same twenty-four-hour period. Patients taking MAO inhibitors should use sumatriptan cautiously.

When these specific abortive medications have not been helpful, patients may respond to acute doses of antinausea medicines, sedatives, cortisone in the form of Decadron, stronger analgesics, opiates, and Stadol NS.

Sympathomimetic Agents

Midrin is one of the best acute-care medicines for tension-type headache and can also be helpful in migraine. Isometheptene mucate in combination with the analgesic acetaminophen and the sedative dichloralphenazone is a very effective agent. For older children and adults, we generally prescribe two capsules, repeated in an hour if necessary, limited to three days per week. Children younger than eighteen years old should start with one capsule.

Like ergotamine, isometheptene mucate is a vasoconstrictor, that is, it combats headache largely by constricting excessively dilated arteries. Midrin does not usually cause or increase nausea as do the ergot compounds and is effective on mild to moderate headache pain. Its side effects are rare and include dizziness and mild sedation, but it is usually very well tolerated.

Other nonergotamine vasoconstrictors include phenylpropanolamine and phenylephrine, available in off-the-shelf headache preparations.

Nonsteroidal Anti-Inflammatory Drugs (NSAIDs)

Both aspirin and ibuprofen (though not Tylenol) fall under this category: drugs that reduce our pain threshold and may keep blood vessels from dilating by inhibiting the production of prostaglandins. There are also over twenty prescription NSAIDs, such as naproxen (Naprosyn), naproxen sodium (Anaprox), meclofenamate (Meclomen), ketoprofen (Orudis), indomethacin (Indocin), and prescription-strength ibuprofen (Motrin).

Nonsteroidal anti-inflammatory drugs are generally prescribed to combat arthritis, which, as pointed out in Chapter 2, sometimes works in the same way as headache does. They may also be used to treat headache, abortively as well as symptomatically. (Some NSAIDs may also at times be used preventively; see below.)

An appropriate dose of a prescription NSAID might be one to two tablets of naproxen or meclofenamate, repeated in one hour if necessary, always with food. We would limit such use of NSAIDs to four tablets three days a week. However, there seems to be some evidence that NSAIDs are less likely than other abortive agents to produce rebound headache. We occasionally prescribe them on a daily basis for short periods of time.

NSAIDs — including aspirin — may accumulate in the kidneys after being used over time. Other possible side effects include edema (swelling) and stomach pain. Most people say they notice no ill effects from NSAIDs, but others have stomach pain or even gastrointestinal bleeding without warning. Always stop taking NSAIDs and call your doctor if you have abdominal pain.

Mixed Barbiturate Analgesics

Some medications contain both an analgesic (such as aspirin or acetaminophen [Tylenol]) and a barbiturate (a sedative such as butalbital). Fiorinal contains aspirin, butalbital, and caffeine; Fioricet contains acetaminophen, butalbital, and caffeine, as does Esgic. Phrenilin and Axocet contain just acetaminophen and butalbital and is better to use before sleep. Axotal is aspirin and butalbital, with no caffeine.

This type of combination drug can be used safely and effectively by the vast majority of headache sufferers if their use is limited to prevent the development of rebound headache. We limit prescriptions to twenty-four tablets a month, without refills. In our opinion, use of two to four tablets three days per week is acceptable and should not cause analgesic rebound.

Opiates (Narcotic Analgesics)

Codeine combined with aspirin, caffeine, and barbiturate (Fiorinal with codeine) or with acetaminophen (Tylenol with codeine) may provide more powerful pain relief but also poses a greater risk of dependency, addiction, and rebound headache. Codeine contains natural alkaloids that dull the brain's ability to perceive pain, which is why codeine is a component of so many prescription pain relievers.

We limit prescription of any opiates (narcotic analgesic) to sixteen tablets per month, often without refills. Opiates such as codeine, oxycodone (Percocet), propoxyphene (Darvon), and meperidine (Demerol) must always be used sparingly and on a nonrefillable basis.

Dilaudid includes natural opiates, while Demerol includes synthetic opiates. They are usually too powerful for regular use.

Darvon (propoxyphene) is a derivative of methadone. It may be sold as Darvon N, which includes aspirin, or Darvocet-N 200, which includes acetaminophen (Tylenol). Although these are all marketed as nonaddictive drugs, recent evidence suggests that they may be otherwise. In our opinion, the nonopiates are just as effective and a great deal cheaper and safer! Save the opiates for an occasional severe headache.

Butorphanol (Stadol NS) is an opiate in the form of a nasal spray that easily can be used at home, especially if you are nauseated or vomiting. It may have less addiction potential than other opiates, works rapidly, and is effective in relieving pain. Side effects may include dizziness, drowsiness, and nausea. One advantage of Stadol is that it does *not* affect blood vessel activity and is safe for people with coronary disease or hypertension. It should always be used at home.

Corticosteroids

Some acute migraine attacks may not be sufficiently treated with ergots or sumatriptan. In some cases, "rescue" medication such as corticosteroids can be used. We use 4 to 6 mg of dexamethasone by mouth, followed in three hours by an additional 2 to 4 mg if necessary. We limit use of this drug to once or twice a month to avoid the multiple serious consequences of frequent long-term use.

Muscle Relaxants

Parafon Forte is composed of acetaminophen plus chlorzoxazone, a centrally acting muscle relaxant. It is considered nonaddictive. Other muscle relaxants include carisoprodol (Soma), cyclobenzaprine (Flexeril), metaxalone (Skelatin), and clonazepam (Klonopin).

New Products

1. *Imitrex (sumatriptan) tablets* were released in September 1995. We have studied it in our Center and it is safe, almost as effective as the injectable form, but will work a bit more slowly. It is available in 25 and 50 mg tablets.
2. *Migranal,* the nasal spray form of D.H.E. 45, is under investigation by the FDA. All studies to date show it to be safe, effective, and easy to use, with rapid relief.
3. *Several experimental tablets and nasal sprays* should become available over the next three to five years and may be very helpful additions to our headache armamentarium.

PREVENTIVE MEDICATION FOR MIGRAINE

Withdrawing from Abortive Medication

Often we find ourselves treating patients who have been overusing analgesic pain relievers or ergotamine compounds, thus setting themselves up for painful, daily, and at times constant rebound headaches. In most cases, our first step is to help the patient reduce her dependence on pain relievers or ergot compounds while helping her switch to preventive medications. Successful treatment of headache is impossible until the excessive use of analgesics is stopped. Our research has shown that simply stopping analgesics often results in a 50 percent decrease in headache frequency and intensity all by itself, in four to six weeks.

Withdrawal from abortive medication may require hospitalization, particularly when a patient is withdrawing from long-term barbiturate, ergotamine, or opiate overuse. This can be a difficult or painful process, but in our opinion, it's clearly worthwhile: Research has shown that almost

90 percent of patients helped to withdraw from overuse of certain medication have a marked reduction in headache, usually within several days.

We treat patients hospitalized at the Greenwich Hospital In-patient Headache Unit with repetitive intravenous D.H.E. 45 after pretreating them with the antinausea drugs promethazine or metoclopramide. Sometimes adjuvant neuroleptic drugs — chlorpromazine (Thorazine) or prochlorperazine (Compazine) — or steroids (dexamethasone or hydrocortisone) can help control headaches during withdrawal. Oral phenobarbital is substituted for the butalbital in Fiorinal, Fioricet, and Esgic. Clonidine can help with withdrawal from opiates (narcotics) by preventing withdrawal reactions such as shaking, diarrhea, and trouble sleeping.

Patients who have been overusing nonprescription medications — salicylates (aspirin) or acetaminophen (Tylenol) — should also be encouraged to discontinue them slowly, over one week. We have used nonsteroidal anti-inflammatory drugs (NSAIDs) such as naproxen sodium (Anaprox) and meclofenamate (Meclomen) to help patients withdraw from aspirin, Tylenol, and combination analgesics. Sometimes the NSAIDs are being abused and need to be withdrawn. Igomethepene (e.g., in Midrin) may be used as a tapering agent as well.

Who Should Take Preventive Medication?

Once a patient has freed herself from reliance on abortive medication, we can explore with her the many types of preventive medications that may help relieve or reduce the frequency, intensity, or duration of her pain. Generally, preventive medication is indicated for patients who have headache attacks three or more times per month, or for those who have one or two prolonged attacks per month but respond slowly or poorly to abortive medications.

If the frequency, duration, and intensity of headache attack are reduced by 50 percent or more, we consider preventive medication worthwhile. Once attacks have been controlled for three to six months, medication can be tapered and eventually discontinued.

It's important to emphasize that preventive medication does not *cure* the headache condition. At best, it simply brings under control the patient's tendency to headache. Biologically speaking, nondrug approaches to headache may bring that tendency under control in exactly the same way. That's why we utilize behavioral approaches to help patients reduce and eventually eliminate their reliance on preventive medication.

Following are the main categories of preventive medications, their effects, and side effects.

Beta-Blockers

Beta-blockers are the most widely used class of drugs for the prevention of migraine. They are 60 to 70 percent effective in producing a greater-than-50-percent reduction in attack frequency.

No one is sure exactly how beta-blockers work. Apparently they act on the brain centers that regulate blood vessel activity, as well as affecting the blood vessels themselves. They may prevent vessels from dilating and reduce the brain's sympathetic tone. They may also affect the body's production of noradrenaline as well as its use of serotonin, the neurotransmitter that, as described in Chapter 2, is deeply involved in migraine, depression, sleep, and a sense of well-being.

Inderal (propranolol) is the most popular type of beta-blocker, used to treat migraine as well as high blood pressure (to which many migraineurs are also prone). Some doctors prescribe it for angina pectoris, arrhythmia, and tremor. Nadolol (Corgard), atenolol (Tenormin), timolol (Blocadren), and metoprolol (Lopressor) are other effective beta-blockers.

Some beta-blockers are long-acting, while others work only for six to eight hours; hence, dosage varies considerably, and scheduling may range from once per day to several times daily. However, you should always begin with the lowest possible dose, increasing your medication only as you and your doctor evaluate your response.

The relative efficacy of the different beta-blockers has not been established, so you and your doctor's choice of which beta-blocker is right for you will depend on a variety of factors. You may need some time for trial and error to hit upon the right beta-blocker in the right dosage for your particular condition. Generally, a beta-blocker should be given a trial period of six to eight weeks.

Our three favorite beta-blockers are nadolol (Corgard), starting at 20 mg each morning; atenolol (Tenormin), starting at 25 mg each morning, and propranolol (Inderal), in a starting dose of 10 mg three times per day. Doses are raised every seven to fourteen days until an effective dose is reached.

People with congestive heart failure, asthma, or insulin-dependent diabetes should not be given the so-called non-selective beta-blockers (e.g., nadolol, propranolol, timolol) but should use the selective ones instead (atenolol, metoprolol, and acebutolol).

As with many medications, beta-blockers' effectiveness may decrease over time, requiring ever-higher dosages — another reason to work toward a switch to drug-free approaches, even if the beta-blockers are working well.

The side effects of beta-blockers include a lower tolerance for exercise, fatigue, depression, increased cholesterol levels, weight gain, and increased susceptibility to hypoglycemia (see Chapter 7). Some people suffer decreased sexual appetite, hair loss, or gastrointestinal distress. Others experience loss of memory, or an inability to concentrate.

These effects are all reversible by lowering the dose or withdrawing the drug completely. If you've been taking high doses, it may take you a while to free yourself from any possible negative effects. The drug should not be stopped suddenly but tapered gradually to prevent rebound headache, rapid heart beat, or tremors. You may not immediately recognize the side effects of beta-blockers as resulting from the drug, since many headache sufferers are prone to depression, weight gain, and high cholesterol levels. High cholesterol may be inherited or related to poor diet and lack of exercise, but can be made worse by treatment with beta-blockers.

Calcium Channel Blockers

This preventive medication keeps calcium ions from crossing the membranes into the muscle cells in the arterial wall, thus preventing vasoconstriction and spasms of the blood vessel. Doctors reason that if vasoconstriction is prevented, the first phase of migraine will not follow; therefore, the migraine process is stopped before it can begin. There is some recent research suggesting that calcium channel blockers may prevent the early stages of migraine, including visual aura, possibly via their effect in brain cells. This medication has *no* effect on the rest of the body's use of calcium, and it is often prescribed for other conditions, such as hypertension, poor circulation, and some gastrointestinal problems, as well as headache.

Major calcium channel blockers include verapamil (Calan, Isoptin), diltiazem (Cardizem), nifedipine (Procardia), and nicardipine (Cardene). Unfortunately, flunarazine, the calcium channel blocker with the best-documented efficacy in migraine prevention, is not available in the United States. Verapamil is the most commonly used drug available in this country; research suggests that nifedipine (Procardia) may be less effective, as it causes too much dilation of blood vessels and occasionally increases headache. Another calcium channel blocker, nimodipine (Nimotop) seems to work better for cluster headache, but can help in migraine and, like Cardene, acts more specifically on cerebral vessels.

Patients who suffer from migraine with aura and those who suffer from cluster headache may benefit from calcium channel blockers more than patients who have migraine without aura. Apparently, chances for benefit from this type of drug increase as the patient continues to take it, so that at least a two-month trial period should be attempted.

Side effects include low blood pressure, swollen ankles, dizziness, nausea, and constipation. There are preliminary reports that it reduces the sperm's penetration of the egg and may therefore reduce male fertility. It should not be used if you have severe heart disease.

Serotonin-Receptor Antagonists

Methysergide maleate (Sansert) is one of the oldest and most effective medications used to prevent migraine. It is an ergot derivative that seems to constrict blood vessels, as well as work to inhibit serotonin$_2$ receptor sites in the brain. It has a beneficial effect on serotonin receptors, which decreases the frequency of migraine. It is one of only three medications approved by the FDA as a preventive for migraine. Some 50 to 60 percent of the migraineurs who have tried methysergide find that it brings some relief.

Because of the potential side effects of this drug — excess accumulation of connective tissue (fibrosis) around abdominal organs, the lungs, and the heart — methysergide is not usually considered a "frontline measure." Its other side effects include stomach pains, muscle aches, leg or chest pain, difficulty sleeping, and possibly hallucinations.

Nevertheless, methysergide is usually quite safe — at its typical dosage of 2 mg three times per day — if "drug holidays" are given periodically. Ideally, methysergide should only be used for five to six months at a time, followed by a four-week period without medication. When we need to investigate the presence of an overgrowth of connective tissue, we do an electrocardiogram, chest X ray, and kidney

X ray (intravenous pyelogram, or IVP) or magnetic resonance imaging (MRI) scan and blood tests of kidney function. The process of stopping the drug must be carefully monitored; it should never be terminated abruptly but must be tapered off over several days so as to avoid a rebound headache.

Another serotonin$_2$ receptor antagonist is cyproheptadine (Periactin), an antihistamine that, like methysergide, prevents migraine by acting at serotonin receptor sites in the brain. Further, like calcium channel blockers, cyproheptadine prevents calcium from passing through the cell membranes and entering the muscle cells in the wall of the blood vessel, helping to prevent arterial spasm.

This drug seems especially helpful for those women with menstrual migraine. It can also be used to combat headaches resulting from withdrawal from estrogen supplements or birth control pills, as it tends to stabilize blood vessels. Given a one- to two-month trial, it may prove very effective in decreasing headaches to one or fewer per month, after which it can be eliminated altogether. The starting dose is one-quarter of a 4 mg tablet one to two hours before bedtime. This can be slowly raised to one to two tablets.

The main side effects of Periactin are a tendency to weight gain, an increased appetite, dry mouth, and drowsiness in the morning. It usually helps sleep. It is our first choice as a preventive medication for children with migraine, and they usually do not experience side effects. It is contraindicated in people with glaucoma and prostatic enlargement.

Finally, methylergonovine maleate (Methergine) is chemically related to methysergide and is also a vasoconstrictor that blocks serotonin receptors. It has replaced ergonovine, an ergot alkaloid no longer commercially available. The dose is 0.2 mg three times per day. It may be helpful even when Sansert is not. Side effects include muscle cramps; chest pain is a rare but significant side effect.

Antidepressants

Antidepressants are often the drugs of choice in patients with chronic daily headache, but they may also be useful in migraine — especially if the patient has a sleep disturbance and/or coexisting depression. The biochemistry of migraine, sleep disorder, and depression is similar and may be related to low levels of the neurotransmitter serotonin.

Antidepressants were designed to treat depression, but they may provide nondepressed headache-prone sufferers relief from headache with no noticeable change in emotions — suggesting that migraine and depression are inherited together on the same chromosome and that increased serotonin levels may treat both conditions. The frequent coexistence of two medical conditions is known as "comorbidity."

There are several different types of antidepressants: *tricyclics, tetracyclics, specific serotonin-reuptake inhibitors,* and *monoamine oxidase (MAO) inhibitors.*

Tricyclics Some of these antidepressants have been available for many years. As discussed in Chapter 2, levels of serotonin may be involved in a person's tendency to headache. These medications prevent serotonin from being reabsorbed into the nerve terminals, thereby increasing its level in the brain and making it more effective. Higher — or possibly more stable — serotonin levels seem to prevent headache, alleviate depression, and contribute to undisturbed sleep. The neurotransmitter noradrenaline can also help to treat headache and depression, and its level is increased by certain tricyclics.

An oft-prescribed tricylic is amitriptyline HCl (Elavil, Endep). It has been a mainstay of pain and headache therapy for thirty years. Others in this class include nortriptyline HCl (Pamelor), doxepin HCl (Sinequan, Adapin), and imipramine (Tofranil). Generally, the tricyclics are useful in treating both migraine and chronic daily headache; they may also work well when combined with a beta-blocker or calcium channel blocker.

You and your doctor may need to explore the effects of various types of tricyclics, as their side effects may include lower blood pressure, weight gain, a dry mouth, trouble urinating, constipation, blurred vision, intense dreams, sexual dysfunction, and sedation.

Tricyclics should not be taken by anyone with a severe disturbance of heart rhythm or a recent heart attack, epilepsy, some forms of glaucoma, and significant enlargement of the prostate gland. Anyone who is already taking medications that cause sedation should discuss with her doctor the possible combined effects of these medications and tricyclics before beginning treatment.

At The New England Center for Headache, we tend to use amitriptyline (Elavil), nortriptyline (Pamelor), doxepin (Sinequan), and trazodone (Desyrel) — which belongs in a miscellaneous category — especially when there is a coexisting sleep problem like waking too early and not being able to get back to sleep. Nortriptyline tends to alert patients more during the day, as does desipramine (Norpramin). The most alerting is protriptyline (Vivactil), usually given in the morning because of its stimulating qualities. All of these medications need to be given for two to four weeks before benefit can be seen. The usual starting dose is one tablet of the smallest dose available, which is often 10 mg but could be 25 or 50 mg, depending on the agent. Doxepin is started at 10 mg at about 8:00 P.M. and raised every five to seven days until a dose of 50 mg is reached. Patients may have more side effects the first few days of usage, but they tend to adapt to them over the first week or two. The exact dose varies for each individual. Some of the medications can be followed by obtaining therapeutic blood levels, but this is usually not necessary. Nortriptyline is one of the few drugs with a "narrow therapeutic window" (too much or too little will be ineffective), so occasional blood levels should be checked.

Tetracyclics The efficacy of the tetracyclics as a treatment for headache has not yet been documented. A key tetracyclic is maprotiline (Ludiomil), starting at 25 mg before sleep. It helps people to sleep through the night.

Specific Serotonin-Reuptake Inhibitors As the name suggests, drugs in this category affect the nerve's ability to take up serotonin; thus, it remains in the synapse longer, raising the concentration of serotonin and increasing its effectiveness. Perhaps the best-known drug in this category is fluoxetine (Prozac). Sertraline (Zoloft), paroxetene (Paxil), and nefazodone (Serzone) are other specific serotonin-reuptake inhibitors. None of these drugs has been established as an effective anti-migraine treatment, although Prozac and Paxil have been reported helpful in chronic tension-type headache.

Certainly Prozac has received an enormous amount of publicity in the last few years. Some people claim that it has made a huge difference in relieving their depression and has changed their lives; others may react with increased sadness, strange feelings, and other disturbing side effects, although this is rare and stops when Prozac is discontinued. It seems able to both cause and relieve headache, depending on the patient, the dose, and the circumstances. An increase in headache occurs in only 10 to 15 percent of patients. We like the drug in patients with chronic daily headache as it is often effective lessening headache, allowing more energy, and having few side effects. It takes four to six weeks to reach therapeutic levels and several weeks to get out of your body once it is stopped. We start with 10 mg at 7:00 A.M. for two weeks and increase to 20 mg at 7:00 A.M. Occasional patients need up to 40 or 60 mg per day. Side effects include weight loss, anxiety, insomnia, tremor, decreased libido, inability to have an orgasm, increased headache, and possible depression. Do not be afraid of it but use only when appropriate and under careful medical supervision. It is the safest antidepressant for patients with heart disease.

Paxil (paroxetene) is started at 10 mg each morning and sertraline (Zoloft) at 25 mg. Paxil can cause nausea for five to ten days and Zoloft can cause gas, diarrhea, and abdominal cramps.

MAO Inhibitors These are an older class of antidepressants, which can interact badly with certain medications and common foods. Patients must observe strict rules about diet and avoid *tyramine* in all its forms (e.g., liver, aged cheese, balsamic vinegar, red wine), and take no cold or pain medications like Sudafed or opiates like Demerol. Tyramine is normally inactivated by monoamine oxidase, and when you are taking Nardil, tyramine ingestion will cause elevated blood pressure.

Side effects of MAO inhibitors include lower or higher blood pressure, diminished interest in sex, weight gain, difficulty sleeping, and dizziness.

The best-known MAO inhibitor is phenelzine (Nardil), which has been used successfully with patients who don't respond well to other measures. Treatment combining MAO inhibitors and certain tricyclics is potentially dangerous but has occasionally proven successful in very refractory patients. The starting dose of Nardil is 15 mg at 7:00 A.M. The dose can be raised weekly up to between 60 to 75 mg per day. When given after noon, it can cause insomnia.

Anticonvulsants

Sometimes drugs used to treat epilepsy — divalproex sodium (Depakote), phenytoin (Dilantin), and carbamazepine (Tegretol) — can also be used to prevent headache.

Most recently, divalproex sodium (Depakote) has been carefully studied as a possible treatment for migraine and cluster headache; it seems to raise GABA (gamma-aminobutyric acid) levels in the brain. GABA inhibits electrical potentials and may help headaches by quieting an electrically irritable migraine brain. Two double-blind, placebo-controlled studies of Depakote have shown significant decreases in migraine headaches. Abbott Laboratories has applied to the FDA for approval of Depakote as a preventive drug for migraine. The starting dose of Depakote is 125 mg twice per day, and the total dose is about 750 mg per day. Blood levels should be checked occasionally, as should your blood count and liver functions. Side effects include weight gain, hair loss, drowsiness, and gastrointestinal problems, but Depakote is generally well-tolerated. It does not affect libido, exercise tolerance, and asthma as do beta-blockers, and should be considered a first-line treatment.

If other medications have failed, and particularly if your EEG (electroencephalogram, a measurement of your brain-wave activity) is abnormal, anticonvulsants may be an effective treatment.

Phenytoin is sometimes successful in the treatment of childhood migraine. Carbamazepine has seen some success in the treatment of cluster headache, as well as in treating patients who don't respond well to any other treatment.

Nonsteroidal Anti-Inflammatory Drugs (NSAIDs)

We've already pointed out that NSAIDs may be used symptomatically or abortively; they may be used preventively as well. Naproxen sodium (Anaprox), meclofenamate (Meclomen), flurbiprofen (Ansaid), ketoprofen (Orudis), and ibuprofen (Advil, Nuprin, Motrin) may be used in this way, particularly to prevent menstrual migraine. They are prescribed with meals. Ketoprofen is available in a long-acting form that bypasses the stomach. It is Oruvail, 200 mg once per day.

Side effects of these drugs include water retention and gastrointestinal symptoms, especially stomach pain and acid reflux. Particular caution is needed with patients older than age 60, in whom gastrointestinal bleeding may occur without pain. If NSAIDs are prescribed over an extended period of time, doctors should monitor kidney function and check for occult (invisible) blood in the stool. We usually prescribe histamine blockers such as Zantac, or Axid, to lower acid secretion and decrease the chance of ulcer. We try at least three different types of NSAIDs before saying they are not helpful.

Miscellaneous Preventive Treatments

Alpha Stimulators Clonidine (Catapres) can help prevent migraine, especially in menopausal women. It can also help in withdrawal from opiates and nicotine. The drug seems to work by decreasing production of adrenaline in the back of the brain in an area called the brain stem. A typical dose is one-half of a 0.1-mg tablet, taken twice per day. The maximum dose is three full tablets spread out over the day. Clonidine is also available as patches that can be worn on the skin — called Catapres TTS #1, #2, and #3 — each containing different amounts of medication. A patch can be worn constantly and needs to be changed only weekly.

The side effects of this medication include dizziness and drowsiness. It decreases blood pressure, but not usually to a dangerously low level. Patients who are on other blood pressure medications or who already feel dizzy or drowsy should not take this drug.

Lithium Lithium carbonate is used mostly to treat cluster headache but on occasion can be given for migraine. Patients who have depression, mania, or mood swings in addition to migraine seem to do better on this drug. It is important to avoid dehydration and increased salt intake when you are taking lithium. We follow drug levels closely. The starting dose is 150 mg twice per day, and it can be raised slowly to a maximum of 300 mg three times per day. It should be taken cautiously with calcium channel blockers and also with

Prozac and diuretics. Side effects include tremor, fatigue, and memory problems.

Stimulant Medications Although not usually used in headache, dextroamphetamine (Dexedrine), methylphenidate (Ritalin), or pemoline (Cylert) may occasionally help to reduce headache. Patients also like the side effects of weight loss and alertness. The usual starting dose of Dexedrine is 5 mg per day, and it can be increased to a total of 20 mg per day. It should not be taken in the afternoon, as it can keep you awake.

TREATMENT OF MENSTRUALLY RELATED HEADACHES

When women have headaches exclusively around their menses (true menstrual migraine) or when they have an increased frequency of headaches in the perimenstrual time, they can be treated with a variety of techniques. We first try to use an anti-inflammatory drug three times per day, starting approximately four days before the start of menses and until the end of menses. The dose is one capsule with each meal; they prevent the formation of prostaglandins by the uterus. This decreases pain and inflammation during menses and possibly also decreases headache. We start with naproxen sodium (Anaprox) or meclofenamate (Meclomen).

As menstrual headaches are thought to be set off by falling levels of beta estradiol prior to the period, we sometimes treat patients by replacing estradiol in the form of Estrace (1 mg per day) or an Estraderm skin patch. This has a 30 to 50 percent chance of markedly reducing menstrually related headaches and does not usually cause side effects.

Other types of hormonal manipulation are tamoxifen (Nolvadex), which is an antiestrogen compound, and danazol (Danocrine), which is an androgen or male hormone. These strong medications drastically change the normal hormonal cycle and should be used only in conjunction with gynecologic consultation.

On occasion acetazolamide (Diamox), a diuretic that decreases the production of spinal fluid, will help decrease menstrual headaches. The starting dose is 125 mg three times per day, and that dose can be doubled.

TRANQUILIZERS

Let us repeat: We do *not* recommend tranquilizers as a long-term approach to headache. Their side effects include dependency, addiction, disorientation, loss of coordination, lack of concentration, drowsiness, weight gain, and depression. Moreover, they may sap your strength and motivation for seeking out drug-free approaches to preventing headaches, approaches that could bring new energy and well-being into your life.

Tranquilizers act primarily as anti-anxiety medication. When taking Valium, women with tension-type headache may benefit from looser muscles, and women with migraine may get fewer headaches, because of the reduction of stress.

In the long run, however, there are plenty of other ways to relax your muscles, ways that bring positive side effects, rather than the negative ones associated with tranquilizers. If you and your doctor are committed to using tranquilizers for a short time, you would do well to set a definite time limit together and make a specific plan for coping with the physical or emotional problems that led to this choice in the first place.

Benzodiazepines (diazepam [Valium], alprazolam [Xanax], chlorazepate [Tranxene], clonazepam [Klonopin], chlordiazepoxide [Librium], lorazepam [Ativan]) all tend to be highly addictive and must be used with extreme care. It may take several months to get off these medications if you have been on them for several months or longer.

Buspirone (BuSpar) is an effective anti-anxiety medication

that is taken on a daily basis and that does not cause dependency or addiction. The starting dose is 5 mg twice per day, but some patients need 60 mg or more.

Phenothiazines (Thorazine) are even stronger than benzodiazepines and are generally considered too strong for headache treatment. We have found, however, that our hospital patients occasionally benefit from using them as a short-term approach to relief of severe headache or nausea and vomiting, rather than using narcotics.

Side effects for this medication include drowsiness, low blood pressure, and dizziness. Long-term use may create a pattern of uncontrollable, spontaneous movements of the face and tongue, known as *tardive dyskinesia*. For a person who already feels out of control of her life, the sense that her muscles are moving "on their own" may be profoundly disturbing. This side effect usually occurs only after high doses are given for many weeks or months.

TREATING TENSION-TYPE HEADACHES

A range of medications are available to treat this headache syndrome:

- *Nonsteroidal anti-inflammatory drugs* may be effective for pain that originates in the neck. These drugs include aspirin, indomethacin (Indocin), naproxen sodium (Anaprox), ibuprofen (Advil, Nuprin, Motrin), or meclofenamate (Meclomen) and others.

- *Tricylic and other types of antidepressants* seem most effective for chronic tension-type headaches (chronic daily headache). Often used for this condition is amitriptyline HCl (Elavil, Endep); nortriptyline NCl (Pamelor), desipramine HCl (Norpramin), or doxepin HCl (Sinequan, Adapin). All other antidepressants on pages 223–226 can be helpful. They are taken at low doses one to two hours before bedtime for several months, with dosages gradually increasing from 10 mg to about 50 mg.

- *Beta-blockers* and *calcium channel blockers* are sometimes used to act on the brain centers that produce chronic daily headache. Generally, however, they are less effective.

- *Muscle relaxants* such as carisoprodol (Soma), cyclobenzaprine (Flexeril), orphenadrine citrate (Norflex), or metaxalone (Skelaxin) may sometimes be prescribed for tension-type headaches, but they should only be used on a short-term basis. They often cause drowsiness.

- *Tranquilizers* may also be prescribed for headache, but we do not recommend them. (See preceding section.) There are many nonpharmacological approaches to the treatment of tension-type headache.

ABORTIVE TREATMENT OF CLUSTER HEADACHE

The best treatment for cluster headache is placing a loose-fitting mask over your nose and mouth and breathing pure oxygen at seven liters per minute for about fifteen minutes. This should be done in a seated position, bending forward. In addition, ergotamine tartrate can be given in the form of Cafergot by mouth or under the tongue, or by rectal suppository to stop an attack. Dihydroergotamine (D.H.E. 45) can be injected in a dose of 1 mg intramuscularly, subcutaneously, or intravenously to stop a cluster headache. The soon-to-be-released nasal spray called Migranal should be very helpful. Subcataneous sumatriptan (Imitrex) has not yet been approved by the FDA for treatment of acute cluster headache. However, the literature indicates that it rapidly stops cluster headache, according to a report from Scandinavia. Cluster patients often turn to the use of daily opiates because their head pain is so severe. Some respond to cocaine sprayed into the back of the nose. Lidocaine nose drops have sometimes been successful. Capsaicin (an extract of red peppers) in the form of off-the-shelf Zostrix HP (0.075 percent) can also help to decrease the severity of the pain.

PREVENTIVE TREATMENT OF CLUSTER HEADACHE

There are multiple medications that can be tried to prevent cluster headache. Verapamil and other calcium channel blockers are safe and effective and have very few side effects. The average dose is 80 mg three times per day, and the maximum dose is usually 160 mg three times a day. The major side effects are constipation and fluid retention. Cluster-headache patients need higher doses than migraineurs.

High-dose steroid treatment by mouth can be very helpful in stopping cluster-headache attacks. The usual dose is 40 to 60 mg of prednisone per day, gradually decreased over two to three weeks. Most patients may get some minor side effects but do not mind them because of the relief from the severity of the cluster attack. Patients can take ergotamine tartrate (Cafergot) tablets on a preventive basis by taking one tablet in the morning and one at night. Sometimes the caffeine in the nighttime dose may keep people awake.

Lithium carbonate can be very helpful in certain patients with cluster headache. The usual dose is 150 mg twice per day and can be brought up to 600 to 900 mg per day. Blood levels should be watched carefully, and patients should be advised not to become dehydrated, take diuretics, or use much verapamil.

Methysergide (Sansert) is a good vasoconstrictor and serotonin$_2$ blocker that works to prevent cluster headache as well as migraine. It should be given as a 2 mg tablet three times a day. Divalproex sodium (Depakote) seems to work in some patients with cluster headache. The starting dose is 125 mg two times per day and can be gradually raised to 750 mg per day.

Indomethacin (Indocin) can help cluster-headache patients at a dose of 25 to 50 mg three times per day with meals.

Acetazolamide (Diamox) can sometimes be helpful in patients with cluster headache.

Several experimental studies have demonstrated the effectiveness of capsaicin, an extract of red peppers, in the form of Zostrix. It should be applied two times per day to the inside of the nostril on the side of the pain. After five to seven days the burning from the capsaicin stops and then the pain from the cluster headache usually decreases or stops.

When none of the above techniques have been helpful, patients may need to take opiates. Our preference is butorphanol nasal spray (Stadol NS), which can be taken as 1 mg doses (one spray in one nostril).

Some patients need to be treated on an inpatient basis. We admit them to the Greenwich Hospital Inpatient Headache Unit. The success rate in episodic cluster headache is extremely high. The success rate in chronic cluster headache is somewhat lower, with most patients doing very well in the hospital but sometimes relapsing after discharge.

If patients have chronic paroxysmal hemicrania, a variant of cluster headache in which each attack lasts for only five to twenty minutes and occurs twelve to fifteen times per day, they will probably respond well to indomethacin (Indocin) at doses of 25 mg three times per day.

AN APPROACH TO USING MEDICATION

Did you know that sometimes *stopping* medication can bring relief from pain? Our own studies have shown that if people with chronic daily headache are dependent on analgesics, and they stop taking those analgesics with no other treatment, 50 percent do at least 50 percent better after the first month. A full 85 percent do at least 50 percent better after three months. This improvement isn't mysterious or "psychological"; it occurs because the *analgesic rebound effect* has been addressed. Far from relieving pain, these medications were actually causing it.

You, too, may need to consider with your doctor how your patterns of taking medication have affected you. If you've been taking barbiturates, opiates (narcotics), ergots, tranquilizers, or sedatives, you should discuss ways of withdrawing from these drugs. You certainly shouldn't try to stop all medication on your own without first discussing it with your doctor! You may need supervision or even hospitalization to help you make the transition, particularly if you suffer from cardiac disease, hypertension, diabetes, depression, or anxiety. It's possible to make withdrawal safe and relatively painless, if you and your doctor work together.

Off-the-shelf medications, on the other hand, pose no dangers from withdrawal — but you may find that it's difficult to stop taking them if you're used to turning to them for headache relief. We often suggest that vitamin B_6 or the antihistamine cyproheptadine (Periactin) be taken to ease the headache pain that initially results from stopping pain medication. We also prescribe Midrin, antinausea medication, a mild sedative, or anti-inflammatory drugs to help you through this time.

Withdrawal in this case may be difficult, but it's definitely worth it; once you've freed yourself from dependence on pain medication, you're likely to feel less pain and fewer unwanted side effects. We conducted a study of sixty-nine women and twenty-one men who stopped taking analgesic medication: *82 percent were getting at least two-thirds fewer headaches within four months!*

Whether you're concerned about withdrawal or simply

following your doctor's prescription, we urge you to work closely with your doctor. For medication to be effective, it's essential that the two of you develop a relationship in which he or she is familiar with how a medication is affecting not only your physical well-being but also your life. If you find yourself feeling happier, more in control, better able to make effective and satisfying decisions, then you and your doctor can rest assured that your treatment is proceeding well. If, on the other hand, you find yourself feeling listless, despairing, or becoming low in energy, we urge you to share that emotional reality with your doctor — just as you would tell him or her about any physical side effects you might notice. A good doctor wants to know how medication is affecting not just the symptom but also the whole person that he or she is treating.

COPING WITH HEADACHES: A FINAL WORD

As you can see, there are multiple medications for each type of headache. It is up to the doctor and patient together to find the appropriate combination of nonpharmacologic and pharmacologic techniques for each patient. Although the above information may seem straightforward and easy to follow, the fine-tuning of medication usage can be difficult to convey.

We hope this book has helped you better understand your headaches, your doctor, and yourself. In the final analysis, your own awareness of your body and your emotions, your commitment to your health and your life, and your willingness to heal yourself make the greatest difference in finding an effective headache treatment that works for you. The good news is that it is almost always possible to find *relief from headache* when you go about it the right way. *Good luck on* your journey.

APPENDIX

THE NEW ENGLAND CENTER FOR HEADACHE
HEADACHE CALENDAR

#1 Mild Headache
#2 Moderate-Severe
#3 Incapacitating

Name

Month   Year

	01	02	03	04	05	06	07	08	09	10	11	12	13	14	15	16	17	18	19	20	21	22	23	24	25	26	27	28	29	30	31
Morning																															
Afternoon																															
Evening																															
Sleeptime																															
Medication																															

Relief 0-1-2-3   (0)-none, (1)-slight relief, (2)-moderate relief, (3)-complete relief

TRIGGERS:

Periods:

Index